THIS
Journal Belongs To:

_____

This journal will help you with Intermittent Fasting. Here, you can keep track of calories, macronutrients, fasting times, fasting hours, sleep quality and quantity, workouts, food cravings, and energy levels. There is no "one way" to intermittently fast. We'll discuss the different Intermittent Fasting methods, as well as strategies to help you get started if you are new to this. Intermittent Fasting (also referred to as IF) can sometimes be a little challenging for some, especially in the beginning, but this journal will help you to be more consistent and successful with it.

Intermittent Fasting is used by many for different reasons.

Some use IF to decrease the calories they eat each day so they can lose weight using the "CICO" method (Calories In, Calories Out). By fasting and not eating for part of the day, you naturally decrease calories, put yourself in a calorie deficit and can lose weight. If you start eating at noon and stop eating at 8pm at night, you basically skip breakfast, which, if you eat the same amount of calories you'd normally have for lunch and dinner only, you can achieve a calorie deficit and lose weight. For example, if you normally eat 800 calories each for lunch and dinner, and 600 calories for breakfast, by skipping breakfast, you cut out 600 calories a day, or 4200 calories a week, which will hopefully result in weight loss for you.

To find out how many calories you need to eat each day in order to lose weight, you can visit this website: https://www.freedieting.com/calorie-calculator (this website even has suggested meal plans that you can incorporate into your intermittent fasting routine).

Some people also practice IF as a way to achieve better health. Some studies show that autophagy happens when you fast. In very simple terms, autophagy is a cellular cleanup process the body engages in during intermittent fasting and during exercising. Autophagy is what causes cells to recycle themselves into healthier cells. This also helps to cleans up cell waste, so cell waste doesn't accumulate and lead to disease. Autophagy literally means "self-eating". All of this helps our cells to become more resilient and to work more efficiently.

As you start intermittent fasting, you have a few choices about which protocol you can follow. Here are five of them for you to learn more about:

The 16/8 Protocol

The first intermittent fasting protocol you might want to consider is called the 16/8, or LeanGains. With a 16/8 fasting protocol, you'll fast for 16 hours and eat for 8 hours. This is one of the easier methods of fasting and eating, due to its simplicity and because you don't go as long while fasting. If you fast from 8pm until noon the following day, which is the most common timeframe to follow a 16/8 protocol, you'll also fast while you're sleeping, which can make it a little easier to follow. Depending on circumstances and health situations, some start off their intermittent fasting protocol so they fast for shorter periods of time (14/10, for example, where one fasts for 14 hours and eats for 10 hours) and some will go on to fast for longer periods of time (18/6 or a 20/4 protocol).

One Meal A Day (OMAD) Protocol

This is a fasting protocol where one eats one "meal" during a short period each day. Many follow the OMAD protocol by eating their daily intake of food during one hour per day. Generally, when people follow this protocol, their meal is very hearty and ample enough to get them through until the next day's OMAD period. Some people start out with a 16/8 fasting protocol and then work their way up to the OMAD strategy. Others might only practice OMAD fasting a few days a week, and then use a more lenient fasting strategy on the other days.

The Eat-Stop-Eat IF Protocol

Also called the 24-hour fast, the Eat-Stop-Eat protocol requires you to go a full 24 hours during the fasting periods. You can either do this once or twice per week, so if you are just starting out, you might want to stick to doing it once a week. All you have to do is follow your normal diet the other 6 days of the week, then have one fasting day where you don't eat or drink anything with calories. Just like all other protocols for intermittent fasting, that 24 hours should only include water, coffee, and tea, without anything added to them, such as cream or sugar. This can start when you wake up, and end the following day, or you can choose a starting and ending time in the middle of the day. This is often when people prefer to do it, otherwise you're going over 24 hours.

The Alternate Day Protocol

Another way you can practice IF is by fasting every other day. This is often referred to as an alternate day fasting protocol. There are many different versions of this, so feel free to experiment with it until you figure out what works best for you. For example, you may do 16:8 fasting protocols every other day, or do a full 24 hours fasting every other day. Some people plan their fasting days so they consume absolutely nothing but water and coffee, while others allow about 500 calories during the fasting days. Just remember to pick something that is sustainable for you and will work with your schedule.

The 5:2 Diet Protocol

The 5:2 diet is one where you eat your normal diet for 5 days out of the week, then fast the other 2 days. This is very similar to the 24-hour diet since the 2 fasting days are separated by at least one eating day in between them. However, you do want to eat about 500-600 calories on the fasting days.

Now that we've learned about some different intermittent fasting methods, here are the Do's and Don'ts for IF.

DO: Transition Slowly

Make sure you are not going into intermittent fasting without planning ahead of time, and without really researching different protocols. To find a suitable intermittent fasting protocol, reread the above information, pick a strategy that you think will work well for you and start it. You can change the strategy later if you need to.

For example, if you were to start the 16/8 protocol, you could start doing this protocol a couple days a week instead of every day. Or you can start out by fasting just 12 hours a day at first, then gradually work your way up to 16 hours of fasting per day.

DO: Listen to Your Body

It's vital to listen to your body when you start intermittent fasting. If one strategy isn't working well for you, start a new strategy to see if it works better for you. If you're feeling tired while you fast, you might increase calories, or if you're eating low carb, you might add more carbs to your diet to see if either of these things help increase your energy levels.

Or…if you're not losing weight, you might decrease calories. Start off with a little bit of a calorie decrease at a time and wait a week or two before you decrease calories again. Also, women will specifically want to pay attention to any adverse hormonal changes, such as hair loss, trouble sleeping and missed periods (please see the additional information for women at the end of this intro to intermittent fasting). If any of these things occur, you should add more calories or carbs into your diet to see if you can reverse the adverse hormonal changes. You might also want to visit your Dr or GP to have bloodwork done to look at your hormone levels. Too few calories or a low carbohydrate intake can sometimes negatively affect female hormones.

DO: Stay Hydrated While Fasting

Make sure you're staying hydrated while you fast. People often forget to drink water just because they are fasting and can't consume food or drinks with calories in them. You should also avoid any drinks that might cause you to become dehydrated, like diet sodas. And if you get tired of water, you can drink plain tea or black coffee instead. Also, if you have any signs of an electrolyte imbalance, like dizziness, light-headedness, or a headache, increase electrolytes during your fasting period. Some people drink pickle juice for more electrolytes.

DO: Take Your Schedule Into Consideration

This is an important part of the planning stage as you figure out what type of IF schedule to follow. For example, if there's no way you can have all your meals in just 8 hours because of a crazy schedule, then the 16:8 protocol probably won't be the best for you. Think about your preferences, schedule, and whether or not it will affect others you live with when deciding which one is going to be the best fit. This makes that transition much easier to handle.

DON'T: Make Yourself Uncomfortable

Intermittent fasting can be hard on your body at first, especially if you are used to eating 6-8 small meals throughout the day, or even 3 larger meals a day. This is another reason why you might do better transitioning to eating less meals during the day, then switching up the hours so you are following an intermittent fasting regimen. If you feel like you are faint from going too long without eating, then it is time to re-think the protocol you are following for IF.

DON'T: Start Binge Eating

This is one of the bigger mistakes people make when they first start intermittent fasting. You might find that during the short window when you can eat, all you want to do is binge eat and go for *anything* you can get your hands on. This is the wrong way to fast. Intermittent fasting is not meant to encourage unhealthy eating habits, like binge-eating. Your eating window is not a free-for-all with food. You should eat the same healthy foods you normally would eat within the eating window you follow. If you're having a hard time controlling binge eating, please see your Dr or GP to ask about any help he or she can give you with that.

DON'T: Watch the Clock

While you *do* want to be sure you are waiting the appropriate amount of time while fasting, don't let it take over your life. You want to develop a different mindset with food and how often you should eat, so try to just set a timer on your phone or watch when it's time to eat again. When I fast, I use the Bodyfast app on my phone. I set it to the times I want to fast and eat and when it's time to eat (and stop eating), an alarm on my phone alerts me. You can find it at this website: https://www.bodyfast.de/

Tips for Starting Intermittent Fasting

Here are a few quick tips that can make this transition easier for you, especially if you're new to Intermittent Fasting:

Plan First. Pick your protocol first, then do plenty of planning. You want to make sure you know when you'll eat, what to eat, and how much to eat. You can use this book to track calories, macros and other numbers. There are even some pages included that help you with menu planning.

Start Slow. Don't go extreme on the first day. It's best to start with the lesser protocols, like a 12/12 or 16/8 where you still have a pretty lengthy window of eating. Wait a bit before you go to the OMAD or 24-hour fasting protocols.

Listen to your body. The intermittent fasting method you're using might not work well for you, so if you notice negative side effects, go back to your normal way of eating or a less strict IF protocol.

Consider fasting more in the morning – With an 8-hour eating window, you can choose to schedule it during any time, then fast for the following 16 hours. If you tend to munch at night or like going out with friends in the evenings, you might be better off starting your fast later in the day, then skipping breakfast and eating a late lunch the following day.

"Does this break my fast?" – Anything you eat that contains calories will break your fast. This includes creamer in your coffee and Bulletproof coffee. If you're feeling faint or ill, or you just like flavored coffee, a little creamer in your cuppa or cup of broth won't hurt you, but it's really better to stick to no calories. Also, caffeine can help suppress appetite, so if it's appropriate, you can drink black coffee, plain tea, or diet soda during your fasting periods.

Eat as Healthy as You Can – First of all, you have the freedom to eat whatever you want when you break your fast. However, eating whole, fresh foods will help to keep you more satiated during your eating windows, because these foods tend to contain more fiber, which fills you up (and fiber is also great for your digestion). And of course, fruits, veggies, and other whole foods have vitamins and minerals that your body needs for optimal health. Some people choose to follow a less strict approach to eating, such as eating 80% healthy foods and 20% unhealthy foods (80/20 eating style). How you eat is your choice.

IIFYM (If It Fits Your Macros) – This is another eating strategy some follow during their eating windows. They calculate how many grams of carbs, protein and fats they need in order to support their bodies in a calorie deficit. Then they plan their eating periods around meals that provide the macros they need. With this eating strategy, macros are the focus, so you can eat anything you want, as long as you eat the macros you need during your eating window. This gives people more flexibility with foods they eat. It makes it easier for some to follow specific diets, such as a Vegan diet or Paleo diet. Some people will eat more refined, processed foods and some eat more whole, fresh foods using the IIFYM eating method.

Intermittent Fasting – Specifically for Women

Intermittent fasting is generally safe for most adults. However, there are a few things for women to consider before starting an intermittent fasting plan.

There Are Benefits to Intermittent Fasting

The primary benefit of intermittent fasting is weight loss and fat loss. When you lose weight, your "bad" cholesterol and triglycerides can decrease. You might also decrease you chance of getting certain types of cancers, lower your blood pressure, have better mobility, decrease your risk of heart disease, have less joint pain, improve your blood sugar levels, decrease your chance of getting diagnosed with type 2 diabetes, have a better hormonal balance, improve your sleep apnea symptoms, have better sleep, have a better sex life, improve your self-esteem, have more energy and SO much more! Yes, there are definitely some great reasons to lose weight, especially if you are obese.

If you're doing intermittent fasting due to the benefits of autophagy, you will experience better health at a cellular level, which will help you to experience increased health and energy.

Adverse Hormonal Changes & the Signs You Need to Watch For

While there are many benefits to intermittent fasting and weight loss, if you don't get enough calories or enough of certain macros, like carbohydrates, you may experience some negative hormonal changes. These changes could be due to increased stress, as well. Or your menstrual cycle.

Some changes to look out for are excessive hair loss, a late, irregular or missing period, low energy, bad mood, depression, anxiety, excessive muscle twitching, body pain, more allergic reactions to foods, increased headaches/migraines, water retention, and bloating.

If negative hormonal changes occur, make sure you consult your doctor or GP in case the hormonal changes are signs of a more serious health problem. Evaluate the amount of calories you're eating each day and consider increasing them to see if that helps your symptoms. And, make sure you aren't over-exercising, as that can affect hormones adversely. Last, make sure you get enough sleep at night.

Should I Do Intermittent Fasting While Pregnant or Breastfeeding?

Don't do intermittent fasting while you're pregnant. Pregnancy is *not* the time to focus on losing weight. Eat regular, wholesome meals and snacks, get plenty of rest, walk, and work on growing a beautiful baby. There's plenty of time to lose weight after the baby comes.

If you want to practice intermittent fasting while exclusive breastfeeding, please ask your Dr or GP first. Sometimes, eating a lower amount of calories can decrease your milk supply and you want to make sure your baby is well-fed and nourished. If you can't IF while you breastfeed, you can just eat a little less each day to decrease calories. Getting your baby out on walks is helpful too and will give you and the baby fresh air and exercise.

Thank you for purchasing this journal and I hope it's immensely helpful for you!

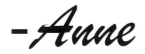

BEFORE & AFTER Pictures

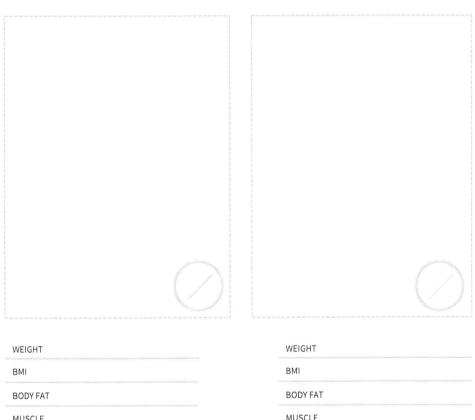

WEIGHT	WEIGHT
BMI	BMI
BODY FAT	BODY FAT
MUSCLE	MUSCLE
CHEST	CHEST
WAIST	WAIST
HIPS	HIPS
THIGHS	THIGHS
CALF	CALF
BICEP	BICEP
OTHER :	OTHER :
OTHER :	OTHER :

WEIGHT LOSS Start Date

Outline your most important fitness goals

Describe how you see yourself in six months

DATE	INTERMITTENT FASTING WEIGHT LOSS ACTION PLAN	PERSONAL MILESTONES

My GO TO **Meals**

BREAKFAST	LUNCH	DINNER	SNACKS

BREAKFAST	LUNCH	DINNER	SNACKS

BREAKFAST	LUNCH	DINNER	SNACKS

BREAKFAST	LUNCH	DINNER	SNACKS

BREAKFAST	LUNCH	DINNER	SNACKS

BREAKFAST	LUNCH	DINNER	SNACKS

BREAKFAST	LUNCH	DINNER	SNACKS

MONTH BY MONTH **Tracker**

JANUARY

FEBRUARY

MARCH

APRIL

MAY

JUNE

MILESTONES

JULY

AUGUST

SEPTEMBER

OCTOBER

NOVEMBER

DECEMBER

NOTES & REFLECTIONS

WEIGHT LOSS **Tracker**

WEEKLY WEIGHT LOSS TRACKER

MONTHLY GOAL

DATE:

	BUST				
	WAIST				
	HIPS				
	BICEP				
	THIGH				
	CALF				
	WEIGHT				
TOTAL WEIGHT LOSS >>					

INTERMITTENT Fasting Log

WEEK OF:

	START TIME	END TIME	TOTAL FAST HRS
M	:	:	:
T	:	:	:
W	:	:	:
T	:	:	:
F	:	:	:
S	:	:	:
S	:	:	:

WEEK OF:

	START TIME	END TIME	TOTAL FAST HRS
M	:	:	:
T	:	:	:
W	:	:	:
T	:	:	:
F	:	:	:
S	:	:	:
S	:	:	:

WEEK OF:

	START TIME	END TIME	TOTAL FAST HRS
M	:	:	:
T	:	:	:
W	:	:	:
T	:	:	:
F	:	:	:
S	:	:	:
S	:	:	:

WEEK OF:

	START TIME	END TIME	TOTAL FAST HRS
M	:	:	:
T	:	:	:
W	:	:	:
T	:	:	:
F	:	:	:
S	:	:	:
S	:	:	:

WEEK OF:

	START TIME	END TIME	TOTAL FAST HRS
M	:	:	:
T	:	:	:
W	:	:	:
T	:	:	:
F	:	:	:
S	:	:	:
S	:	:	:

NOTES & REFLECTIONS

MILESTONES & ACCOMPLISHMENTS

GOALS &
Accomplishments

MONTH | JAN FEB MAR APR MAY JUN JUL AUG SEP OCT NOV DEC

THIS MONTH'S GOALS

ACTION PLAN

M T W T F S S

WEEKLY GOALS

NOTES:

THOUGHTS

MEAL IDEAS:	BREAKFAST	LUNCH	DINNER	SNACKS
M				
T				
W				
T				
F				
S				
S				

MEAL **Planner**

GROCERY LIST

MON

TUES

WED

THUR

FRI

SAT

SUN

My SHOPPING LIST

FRESH PRODUCE

MEAT AND SEAFOOD

DAIRY PRODUCTS

PANTRY ITEMS

FROZEN / OTHER

MY DAILY PROGRESS **Tracker**

SLEEP TRACKER:

DATE _____

RISE: _____

BEDTIME: _____

SLEEP (HRS): _____

NOTES FOR THE DAY

_____

_____

_____

FASTING TIMES & DURATION

EXERCISE / WORKOUT ROUTINE

TOP 6 PRIORITIES OF THE DAY

IN A STATE OF KETOSIS?

YES   NO   UNSURE

WATER INTAKE TRACKER

DAILY ENERGY LEVEL

HIGH   **MEDIUM**   **LOW**

1st MEAL

FAT: CARBS: PROTEIN: CALORIES:

2nd MEAL

FAT: CARBS: PROTEIN: CALORIES:

Other MEALS & SNACKS

FAT: CARBS: PROTEIN: CALORIES:

END OF THE DAY TOTAL OVERVIEW

FAT   CARBS   PROTEIN   KCAL

_____   _____   _____   _____

MY DAILY PROGRESS **Tracker**

SLEEP TRACKER:

DATE _____

RISE: _____   BEDTIME: _____   SLEEP (HRS): _____

NOTES FOR THE DAY

_____
_____
_____

FASTING TIMES & DURATION

EXERCISE / WORKOUT ROUTINE

TOP 6 PRIORITIES OF THE DAY

IN A STATE OF KETOSIS?

YES   NO   UNSURE

WATER INTAKE TRACKER

DAILY ENERGY LEVEL

HIGH   **MEDIUM**   **LOW**

1st MEAL

FAT: CARBS: PROTEIN: CALORIES:

2nd MEAL

FAT: CARBS: PROTEIN: CALORIES:

Other MEALS & SNACKS

FAT: CARBS: PROTEIN: CALORIES:

END OF THE DAY TOTAL OVERVIEW

FAT   CARBS   PROTEIN   KCAL

MY DAILY PROGRESS **Tracker**

SLEEP TRACKER:

DATE _____

RISE: _____

BEDTIME: _____

SLEEP (HRS): _____

NOTES FOR THE DAY

_____

_____

_____

IN A STATE OF KETOSIS?

YES   NO   UNSURE

WATER INTAKE TRACKER

FASTING TIMES & DURATION

DAILY ENERGY LEVEL

HIGH   **MEDIUM**   **LOW**

1st MEAL

FAT: CARBS: PROTEIN: CALORIES:

EXERCISE / WORKOUT ROUTINE

2nd MEAL

FAT: CARBS: PROTEIN: CALORIES:

Other MEALS & SNACKS

FAT: CARBS: PROTEIN: CALORIES:

TOP 6 PRIORITIES OF THE DAY

END OF THE DAY TOTAL OVERVIEW

FAT   CARBS   PROTEIN   KCAL

MY DAILY PROGRESS Tracker

SLEEP TRACKER:

DATE _____

☀ | RISE: | 🌙 z z z | BEDTIME: | 💤 | SLEEP (HRS):

NOTES FOR THE DAY

_____

_____

_____

FASTING TIMES & DURATION

EXERCISE / WORKOUT ROUTINE

TOP 6 PRIORITIES OF THE DAY

○ _____ ○ _____

○ _____ ○ _____

○ _____ ○ _____

IN A STATE OF KETOSIS?

YES   NO   UNSURE

WATER INTAKE TRACKER

DAILY ENERGY LEVEL		
HIGH	**MEDIUM**	**LOW**

1st MEAL

FAT: CARBS: PROTEIN: CALORIES:

2nd MEAL

FAT: CARBS: PROTEIN: CALORIES:

Other MEALS & SNACKS

FAT: CARBS: PROTEIN: CALORIES:

END OF THE DAY TOTAL OVERVIEW

FAT   CARBS   PROTEIN   KCAL

MY DAILY PROGRESS **Tracker**

SLEEP TRACKER:

DATE _____

RISE: _____   BEDTIME: _____   SLEEP (HRS): _____

NOTES FOR THE DAY

_____
_____
_____

FASTING TIMES & DURATION

EXERCISE / WORKOUT ROUTINE

TOP 6 PRIORITIES OF THE DAY

IN A STATE OF KETOSIS?

YES   NO   UNSURE

WATER INTAKE TRACKER

DAILY ENERGY LEVEL

HIGH   **MEDIUM**   **LOW**

1st MEAL

FAT: CARBS: PROTEIN: CALORIES:

2nd MEAL

FAT: CARBS: PROTEIN: CALORIES:

Other MEALS & SNACKS

FAT: CARBS: PROTEIN: CALORIES:

END OF THE DAY TOTAL OVERVIEW

FAT   CARBS   PROTEIN   KCAL

MY DAILY PROGRESS **Tracker**

SLEEP TRACKER:

DATE _____

RISE: _____

BEDTIME: _____

SLEEP (HRS): _____

NOTES FOR THE DAY

_____

_____

_____

IN A STATE OF KETOSIS?

YES   NO   UNSURE

WATER INTAKE TRACKER

FASTING TIMES & DURATION

EXERCISE / WORKOUT ROUTINE

DAILY ENERGY LEVEL

HIGH	MEDIUM	LOW

1st MEAL

FAT:	CARBS:	PROTEIN:	CALORIES:

2nd MEAL

FAT:	CARBS:	PROTEIN:	CALORIES:

Other MEALS & SNACKS

FAT:	CARBS:	PROTEIN:	CALORIES:

TOP 6 PRIORITIES OF THE DAY

END OF THE DAY TOTAL OVERVIEW

FAT	CARBS	PROTEIN	KCAL

MY DAILY PROGRESS **Tracker**

RISE: _____

BEDTIME: _____

SLEEP (HRS): _____

NOTES FOR THE DAY

_____

_____

_____

FASTING TIMES & DURATION

EXERCISE / WORKOUT ROUTINE

TOP 6 PRIORITIES OF THE DAY

○ _____   ○ _____

○ _____   ○ _____

○ _____   ○ _____

IN A STATE OF KETOSIS?

YES   NO   UNSURE

WATER INTAKE TRACKER

DAILY ENERGY LEVEL

HIGH   **MEDIUM**   **LOW**

1st **MEAL**

FAT: CARBS: PROTEIN: CALORIES:

2nd **MEAL**

FAT: CARBS: PROTEIN: CALORIES:

Other **MEALS & SNACKS**

FAT: CARBS: PROTEIN: CALORIES:

END OF THE DAY TOTAL OVERVIEW

FAT   CARBS   PROTEIN   KCAL

MEAL **Planner**

GROCERY LIST

- [ ]
- [ ]
- [ ]
- [ ]
- [ ]
- [ ]
- [ ]
- [ ]
- [ ]
- [ ]
- [ ]
- [ ]
- [ ]
- [ ]
- [ ]
- [ ]
- [ ]

MON

TUES

WED

THUR

FRI

SAT

SUN

My SHOPPING LIST

FRESH PRODUCE

MEAT AND SEAFOOD

DAIRY PRODUCTS

PANTRY ITEMS

FROZEN / OTHER

MY DAILY PROGRESS **Tracker**

SLEEP TRACKER:

DATE _____

RISE: _____   BEDTIME: _____   SLEEP (HRS): _____

NOTES FOR THE DAY

_____

_____

_____

FASTING TIMES & DURATION

EXERCISE / WORKOUT ROUTINE

TOP 6 PRIORITIES OF THE DAY

IN A STATE OF KETOSIS?

YES   NO   UNSURE

WATER INTAKE TRACKER

DAILY ENERGY LEVEL

HIGH   **MEDIUM**   **LOW**

1st MEAL

FAT: CARBS: PROTEIN: CALORIES:

2nd MEAL

FAT: CARBS: PROTEIN: CALORIES:

Other MEALS & SNACKS

FAT: CARBS: PROTEIN: CALORIES:

END OF THE DAY TOTAL OVERVIEW

FAT   CARBS   PROTEIN   KCAL

MY DAILY PROGRESS **Tracker**

DATE

RISE:

BEDTIME:

SLEEP (HRS):

NOTES FOR THE DAY

IN A STATE OF KETOSIS?

YES   NO   UNSURE

WATER INTAKE TRACKER

FASTING TIMES & DURATION

DAILY ENERGY LEVEL		
HIGH	**MEDIUM**	**LOW**

1st MEAL

FAT: CARBS: PROTEIN: CALORIES:

EXERCISE / WORKOUT ROUTINE

2nd MEAL

FAT: CARBS: PROTEIN: CALORIES:

Other MEALS & SNACKS

FAT: CARBS: PROTEIN: CALORIES:

TOP 6 PRIORITIES OF THE DAY

END OF THE DAY TOTAL OVERVIEW

FAT   CARBS   PROTEIN   KCAL

MY DAILY PROGRESS **Tracker**

SLEEP TRACKER:

DATE _____

☼ | RISE:
🌙 zᶻᶻ | BEDTIME:
💤 | SLEEP (HRS):

NOTES FOR THE DAY

_____
_____
_____
_____

IN A STATE OF KETOSIS?

YES   NO   UNSURE

WATER INTAKE TRACKER

FASTING TIMES & DURATION

DAILY ENERGY LEVEL

HIGH	**MEDIUM**	**LOW**

1st **MEAL**

FAT: CARBS: PROTEIN: CALORIES:

2nd **MEAL**

FAT: CARBS: PROTEIN: CALORIES:

EXERCISE / WORKOUT ROUTINE

Other **MEALS** & **SNACKS**

FAT: CARBS: PROTEIN: CALORIES:

TOP 6 PRIORITIES OF THE DAY

○ _____ ○ _____
○ _____ ○ _____
○ _____ ○ _____

END OF THE DAY TOTAL OVERVIEW

FAT   CARBS   PROTEIN   KCAL

_____

MY DAILY PROGRESS **Tracker**

SLEEP TRACKER:

DATE _____

RISE: _____

BEDTIME: _____

SLEEP (HRS): _____

NOTES FOR THE DAY

_____

_____

_____

IN A STATE OF KETOSIS?

YES   NO   UNSURE

WATER INTAKE TRACKER

FASTING TIMES & DURATION

DAILY ENERGY LEVEL

HIGH   **MEDIUM**   **LOW**

1st MEAL

FAT: CARBS: PROTEIN: CALORIES:

EXERCISE / WORKOUT ROUTINE

2nd MEAL

FAT: CARBS: PROTEIN: CALORIES:

Other MEALS & SNACKS

FAT: CARBS: PROTEIN: CALORIES:

TOP 6 PRIORITIES OF THE DAY

END OF THE DAY TOTAL OVERVIEW

FAT   CARBS   PROTEIN   KCAL

MY DAILY PROGRESS **Tracker**

SLEEP TRACKER:

DATE _____

RISE: _____   BEDTIME: _____   SLEEP (HRS): _____

NOTES FOR THE DAY

_____
_____
_____

IN A STATE OF KETOSIS?

YES   NO   UNSURE

WATER INTAKE TRACKER

FASTING TIMES & DURATION

EXERCISE / WORKOUT ROUTINE

DAILY ENERGY LEVEL

HIGH   **MEDIUM**   **LOW**

1st MEAL

FAT: CARBS: PROTEIN: CALORIES:

2nd MEAL

FAT: CARBS: PROTEIN: CALORIES:

Other MEALS & SNACKS

FAT: CARBS: PROTEIN: CALORIES:

TOP 6 PRIORITIES OF THE DAY

END OF THE DAY TOTAL OVERVIEW

FAT   CARBS   PROTEIN   KCAL

MY DAILY PROGRESS **Tracker**

SLEEP TRACKER:

DATE

RISE:

BEDTIME:

SLEEP (HRS):

NOTES FOR THE DAY

IN A STATE OF KETOSIS?

YES   NO   UNSURE

WATER INTAKE TRACKER

FASTING TIMES & DURATION

DAILY ENERGY LEVEL

HIGH   **MEDIUM**   **LOW**

1st MEAL

FAT: CARBS: PROTEIN: CALORIES:

2nd MEAL

FAT: CARBS: PROTEIN: CALORIES:

EXERCISE / WORKOUT ROUTINE

Other MEALS & SNACKS

FAT: CARBS: PROTEIN: CALORIES:

TOP 6 PRIORITIES OF THE DAY

END OF THE DAY TOTAL OVERVIEW

FAT   CARBS   PROTEIN   KCAL

MY DAILY PROGRESS **Tracker**

SLEEP TRACKER:

DATE _____

RISE: _____

BEDTIME: _____

SLEEP (HRS): _____

NOTES FOR THE DAY

_____

_____

_____

FASTING TIMES & DURATION

EXERCISE / WORKOUT ROUTINE

TOP 6 PRIORITIES OF THE DAY

IN A STATE OF KETOSIS?

YES   NO   UNSURE

WATER INTAKE TRACKER

DAILY ENERGY LEVEL		
HIGH	**MEDIUM**	**LOW**

1st MEAL

FAT: CARBS: PROTEIN: CALORIES:

2nd MEAL

FAT: CARBS: PROTEIN: CALORIES:

Other MEALS & SNACKS

FAT: CARBS: PROTEIN: CALORIES:

END OF THE DAY TOTAL OVERVIEW

FAT   CARBS   PROTEIN   KCAL

MEAL Planner

GROCERY LIST

- [ ]
- [ ]
- [ ]
- [ ]
- [ ]
- [ ]
- [ ]
- [ ]
- [ ]
- [ ]
- [ ]
- [ ]
- [ ]
- [ ]
- [ ]
- [ ]
- [ ]
- [ ]

MON

TUES

WED

THUR

FRI

SAT

SUN

My SHOPPING LIST

FRESH PRODUCE

MEAT AND SEAFOOD

DAIRY PRODUCTS

PANTRY ITEMS

FROZEN / OTHER

MY DAILY PROGRESS **Tracker**

SLEEP TRACKER:

DATE _____

RISE: _____ | BEDTIME: _____ | SLEEP (HRS): _____

NOTES FOR THE DAY

_____

_____

_____

FASTING TIMES & DURATION

EXERCISE / WORKOUT ROUTINE

TOP 6 PRIORITIES OF THE DAY

- ○ _____
- ○ _____
- ○ _____
- ○ _____
- ○ _____
- ○ _____

IN A STATE OF KETOSIS?

YES   NO   UNSURE

WATER INTAKE TRACKER

○ ○ ○ ○ ○ ○ ○ ○

DAILY ENERGY LEVEL

HIGH   **MEDIUM**   **LOW**

1ˢᵗ MEAL

FAT: CARBS: PROTEIN: CALORIES:

2ⁿᵈ MEAL

FAT: CARBS: PROTEIN: CALORIES:

Other MEALS & SNACKS

FAT: CARBS: PROTEIN: CALORIES:

END OF THE DAY TOTAL OVERVIEW

FAT   CARBS   PROTEIN   KCAL

____   ____   ____   ____

MY DAILY PROGRESS **Tracker**

SLEEP TRACKER:

DATE _____

☀ RISE: _____   🌙 BEDTIME: _____   💤 SLEEP (HRS): _____

NOTES FOR THE DAY

_____
_____
_____

FASTING TIMES & DURATION

EXERCISE / WORKOUT ROUTINE

TOP 6 PRIORITIES OF THE DAY

○ _____   ○ _____
○ _____   ○ _____
○ _____   ○ _____

IN A STATE OF KETOSIS?

YES   NO   UNSURE

WATER INTAKE TRACKER

DAILY ENERGY LEVEL		
HIGH	**MEDIUM**	**LOW**

1st MEAL

FAT: CARBS: PROTEIN: CALORIES:

2nd MEAL

FAT: CARBS: PROTEIN: CALORIES:

Other MEALS & SNACKS

FAT: CARBS: PROTEIN: CALORIES:

END OF THE DAY TOTAL OVERVIEW

FAT	CARBS	PROTEIN	KCAL

MY DAILY PROGRESS **Tracker**

SLEEP TRACKER:

DATE _____

RISE: _____

BEDTIME: _____

SLEEP (HRS): _____

NOTES FOR THE DAY

_____
_____
_____

FASTING TIMES & DURATION

EXERCISE / WORKOUT ROUTINE

TOP 6 PRIORITIES OF THE DAY

IN A STATE OF KETOSIS?

YES   NO   UNSURE

WATER INTAKE TRACKER

DAILY ENERGY LEVEL

HIGH	**MEDIUM**	**LOW**

1st MEAL

FAT: CARBS: PROTEIN: CALORIES:

2nd MEAL

FAT: CARBS: PROTEIN: CALORIES:

Other MEALS & SNACKS

FAT: CARBS: PROTEIN: CALORIES:

END OF THE DAY TOTAL OVERVIEW

FAT   CARBS   PROTEIN   KCAL

MY DAILY PROGRESS **Tracker**

SLEEP TRACKER:

DATE _____

☼ | RISE: | 🌙 | BEDTIME: | 💤 | SLEEP (HRS):

NOTES FOR THE DAY

_____
_____
_____

FASTING TIMES & DURATION

EXERCISE / WORKOUT ROUTINE

TOP 6 PRIORITIES OF THE DAY

- ○ _____ ○ _____
- ○ _____ ○ _____
- ○ _____ ○ _____

IN A STATE OF KETOSIS?

YES   NO   UNSURE

WATER INTAKE TRACKER

DAILY ENERGY LEVEL

HIGH   **MEDIUM**   **LOW**

1st MEAL

FAT: CARBS: PROTEIN: CALORIES:

2nd MEAL

FAT: CARBS: PROTEIN: CALORIES:

Other MEALS & SNACKS

FAT: CARBS: PROTEIN: CALORIES:

END OF THE DAY TOTAL OVERVIEW

FAT   CARBS   PROTEIN   KCAL

MY DAILY PROGRESS **Tracker**

SLEEP TRACKER:

DATE _____

☀ | RISE: | 🌙 | BEDTIME: | 💭 | SLEEP (HRS): |

NOTES FOR THE DAY

_____

_____

_____

IN A STATE OF KETOSIS?

YES   NO   UNSURE

WATER INTAKE TRACKER

FASTING TIMES & DURATION

DAILY ENERGY LEVEL

| **HIGH** | **MEDIUM** | **LOW** |

1st MEAL

FAT: CARBS: PROTEIN: CALORIES:

EXERCISE / WORKOUT ROUTINE

2nd MEAL

FAT: CARBS: PROTEIN: CALORIES:

Other MEALS & SNACKS

FAT: CARBS: PROTEIN: CALORIES:

TOP 6 PRIORITIES OF THE DAY

- ○ _____ ○ _____
- ○ _____ ○ _____
- ○ _____ ○ _____

END OF THE DAY TOTAL OVERVIEW

FAT   CARBS   PROTEIN   KCAL

MY DAILY PROGRESS **Tracker**

SLEEP TRACKER:

DATE _____

RISE: _____   BEDTIME: _____   SLEEP (HRS): _____

NOTES FOR THE DAY

_____

_____

_____

IN A STATE OF KETOSIS?

YES   NO   UNSURE

WATER INTAKE TRACKER

FASTING TIMES & DURATION

DAILY ENERGY LEVEL		
HIGH	**MEDIUM**	**LOW**

1st MEAL

FAT: CARBS: PROTEIN: CALORIES:

EXERCISE / WORKOUT ROUTINE

2nd MEAL

FAT: CARBS: PROTEIN: CALORIES:

Other MEALS & SNACKS

FAT: CARBS: PROTEIN: CALORIES:

TOP 6 PRIORITIES OF THE DAY

END OF THE DAY TOTAL OVERVIEW

FAT   CARBS   PROTEIN   KCAL

MY DAILY PROGRESS **Tracker**

SLEEP TRACKER:

DATE _____

☀ RISE: _____ 🌙 BEDTIME: _____ 💤 SLEEP (HRS): _____

NOTES FOR THE DAY

_____
_____
_____

FASTING TIMES & DURATION

EXERCISE / WORKOUT ROUTINE

TOP 6 PRIORITIES OF THE DAY

- ○ _____   ○ _____
- ○ _____   ○ _____
- ○ _____   ○ _____

IN A STATE OF KETOSIS?

YES   NO   UNSURE

WATER INTAKE TRACKER

DAILY ENERGY LEVEL

HIGH   **MEDIUM**   **LOW**

1st MEAL

FAT: CARBS: PROTEIN: CALORIES:

2nd MEAL

FAT: CARBS: PROTEIN: CALORIES:

Other MEALS & SNACKS

FAT: CARBS: PROTEIN: CALORIES:

END OF THE DAY TOTAL OVERVIEW

FAT   CARBS   PROTEIN   KCAL

MEAL **Planner**

GROCERY LIST

MON

TUES

WED

THUR

FRI

SAT

SUN

My SHOPPING LIST

FRESH PRODUCE

MEAT AND SEAFOOD

DAIRY PRODUCTS

PANTRY ITEMS

FROZEN / OTHER

MY DAILY PROGRESS **Tracker**

SLEEP TRACKER:

DATE _____

RISE: _____ | BEDTIME: _____ | SLEEP (HRS): _____

NOTES FOR THE DAY

_____

_____

_____

FASTING TIMES & DURATION

EXERCISE / WORKOUT ROUTINE

TOP 6 PRIORITIES OF THE DAY

- ○ _____ ○ _____
- ○ _____ ○ _____
- ○ _____ ○ _____

IN A STATE OF KETOSIS?

YES   NO   UNSURE

WATER INTAKE TRACKER

DAILY ENERGY LEVEL

HIGH   **MEDIUM**   **LOW**

1st MEAL

FAT: CARBS: PROTEIN: CALORIES:

2nd MEAL

FAT: CARBS: PROTEIN: CALORIES:

Other MEALS & SNACKS

FAT: CARBS: PROTEIN: CALORIES:

END OF THE DAY TOTAL OVERVIEW

FAT   CARBS   PROTEIN   KCAL

MY DAILY PROGRESS Tracker

SLEEP TRACKER:

DATE _____

☀ RISE: _____

🌙 z z z BEDTIME: _____

💤 SLEEP (HRS): _____

NOTES FOR THE DAY

_____

_____

_____

FASTING TIMES & DURATION

EXERCISE / WORKOUT ROUTINE

TOP 6 PRIORITIES OF THE DAY

○ _____   ○ _____

○ _____   ○ _____

○ _____   ○ _____

IN A STATE OF KETOSIS?

YES   NO   UNSURE

WATER INTAKE TRACKER

DAILY ENERGY LEVEL

HIGH	MEDIUM	LOW

1st MEAL

FAT: CARBS: PROTEIN: CALORIES:

2nd MEAL

FAT: CARBS: PROTEIN: CALORIES:

Other MEALS & SNACKS

FAT: CARBS: PROTEIN: CALORIES:

END OF THE DAY TOTAL OVERVIEW

FAT	CARBS	PROTEIN	KCAL

MY DAILY PROGRESS **Tracker**

SLEEP TRACKER:

DATE _____

☀ | RISE: _____ | 🌙 zᶻz | BEDTIME: _____ | 💭 | SLEEP (HRS): _____

NOTES FOR THE DAY

_____

_____

_____

FASTING TIMES & DURATION

EXERCISE / WORKOUT ROUTINE

TOP 6 PRIORITIES OF THE DAY

○ _____ ○ _____

○ _____ ○ _____

○ _____ ○ _____

IN A STATE OF KETOSIS?

YES   NO   UNSURE

WATER INTAKE TRACKER

💧 💧 💧 💧 💧 💧 💧 💧

DAILY ENERGY LEVEL

HIGH   **MEDIUM**   **LOW**

1st MEAL

FAT: CARBS: PROTEIN: CALORIES:

2nd MEAL

FAT: CARBS: PROTEIN: CALORIES:

Other MEALS & SNACKS

FAT: CARBS: PROTEIN: CALORIES:

END OF THE DAY TOTAL OVERVIEW

FAT   CARBS   PROTEIN   KCAL

_____   _____   _____   _____

MY DAILY PROGRESS **Tracker**

SLEEP TRACKER:

DATE _____

RISE: _____   BEDTIME: _____   SLEEP (HRS): _____

NOTES FOR THE DAY

_____
_____
_____

FASTING TIMES & DURATION

EXERCISE / WORKOUT ROUTINE

TOP 6 PRIORITIES OF THE DAY

○ _____   ○ _____
○ _____   ○ _____
○ _____   ○ _____

IN A STATE OF KETOSIS?

YES   NO   UNSURE

WATER INTAKE TRACKER

DAILY ENERGY LEVEL

HIGH   **MEDIUM**   **LOW**

1st MEAL

FAT: CARBS: PROTEIN: CALORIES:

2nd MEAL

FAT: CARBS: PROTEIN: CALORIES:

Other MEALS & SNACKS

FAT: CARBS: PROTEIN: CALORIES:

END OF THE DAY TOTAL OVERVIEW

FAT   CARBS   PROTEIN   KCAL

MY DAILY PROGRESS **Tracker**

SLEEP TRACKER:

DATE _____

RISE: _____

BEDTIME: _____

SLEEP (HRS): _____

NOTES FOR THE DAY

_____

_____

_____

FASTING TIMES & DURATION

EXERCISE / WORKOUT ROUTINE

TOP 6 PRIORITIES OF THE DAY

- _____
- _____
- _____
- _____
- _____
- _____

IN A STATE OF KETOSIS?

YES   NO   UNSURE

WATER INTAKE TRACKER

DAILY ENERGY LEVEL

HIGH   **MEDIUM**   **LOW**

1st MEAL

FAT: CARBS: PROTEIN: CALORIES:

2nd MEAL

FAT: CARBS: PROTEIN: CALORIES:

Other MEALS & SNACKS

FAT: CARBS: PROTEIN: CALORIES:

END OF THE DAY TOTAL OVERVIEW

FAT   CARBS   PROTEIN   KCAL

MY DAILY PROGRESS **Tracker**

SLEEP TRACKER:

DATE _____

RISE: _____

BEDTIME: _____

SLEEP (HRS): _____

NOTES FOR THE DAY

_____

_____

_____

FASTING TIMES & DURATION

EXERCISE / WORKOUT ROUTINE

TOP 6 PRIORITIES OF THE DAY

- _____ - _____
- _____ - _____
- _____ - _____

IN A STATE OF KETOSIS?

YES   NO   UNSURE

WATER INTAKE TRACKER

DAILY ENERGY LEVEL

HIGH   **MEDIUM**   **LOW**

1st MEAL

FAT: CARBS: PROTEIN: CALORIES:

2nd MEAL

FAT: CARBS: PROTEIN: CALORIES:

Other MEALS & SNACKS

FAT: CARBS: PROTEIN: CALORIES:

END OF THE DAY TOTAL OVERVIEW

FAT   CARBS   PROTEIN   KCAL

MY DAILY PROGRESS **Tracker**

SLEEP TRACKER:

DATE _____

RISE: _____   BEDTIME: _____   SLEEP (HRS): _____

NOTES FOR THE DAY

_____

_____

_____

IN A STATE OF KETOSIS?

YES   NO   UNSURE

WATER INTAKE TRACKER

FASTING TIMES & DURATION

DAILY ENERGY LEVEL

HIGH	**MEDIUM**	**LOW**

1st MEAL

FAT: CARBS: PROTEIN: CALORIES:

2nd MEAL

FAT: CARBS: PROTEIN: CALORIES:

EXERCISE / WORKOUT ROUTINE

Other MEALS & SNACKS

FAT: CARBS: PROTEIN: CALORIES:

TOP 6 PRIORITIES OF THE DAY

END OF THE DAY TOTAL OVERVIEW

FAT   CARBS   PROTEIN   KCAL

MEAL **Planner**

WEEK OF

GROCERY LIST

MON

TUES

WED

THUR

FRI

SAT

SUN

My SHOPPING LIST

FRESH PRODUCE

MEAT AND SEAFOOD

DAIRY PRODUCTS

PANTRY ITEMS

FROZEN / OTHER

MY DAILY PROGRESS **Tracker**

SLEEP TRACKER:

DATE _____

RISE: _____

BEDTIME: _____

SLEEP (HRS): _____

NOTES FOR THE DAY

_____
_____
_____

FASTING TIMES & DURATION

EXERCISE / WORKOUT ROUTINE

TOP 6 PRIORITIES OF THE DAY

IN A STATE OF KETOSIS?

YES   NO   UNSURE

WATER INTAKE TRACKER

DAILY ENERGY LEVEL

HIGH   **MEDIUM**   **LOW**

1st MEAL

FAT: CARBS: PROTEIN: CALORIES:

2nd MEAL

FAT: CARBS: PROTEIN: CALORIES:

Other MEALS & SNACKS

FAT: CARBS: PROTEIN: CALORIES:

END OF THE DAY TOTAL OVERVIEW

FAT   CARBS   PROTEIN   KCAL

MY DAILY PROGRESS **Tracker**

SLEEP TRACKER:

DATE _____

☀ | RISE: | 🌙 z,z | BEDTIME: | 💭z-z | SLEEP (HRS):

NOTES FOR THE DAY

_____

_____

_____

FASTING TIMES & DURATION

EXERCISE / WORKOUT ROUTINE

TOP 6 PRIORITIES OF THE DAY

○ _____ ○ _____

○ _____ ○ _____

○ _____ ○ _____

IN A STATE OF KETOSIS?

YES   NO   UNSURE

WATER INTAKE TRACKER

DAILY ENERGY LEVEL

HIGH   **MEDIUM**   **LOW**

1st MEAL

FAT: CARBS: PROTEIN: CALORIES:

2nd MEAL

FAT: CARBS: PROTEIN: CALORIES:

Other MEALS & SNACKS

FAT: CARBS: PROTEIN: CALORIES:

END OF THE DAY TOTAL OVERVIEW

FAT   CARBS   PROTEIN   KCAL

WEIGHT LOSS **Tracker**

MONTHLY GOAL

DATE:

BUST					
WAIST					
HIPS					
BICEP					
THIGH					
CALF					
WEIGHT					

TOTAL WEIGHT LOSS >>

INTERMITTENT Fasting Log

	START TIME	END TIME	TOTAL FAST HRS
M	:	:	:
T	:	:	:
W	:	:	:
T	:	:	:
F	:	:	:
S	:	:	:
S	:	:	:

	START TIME	END TIME	TOTAL FAST HRS
M	:	:	:
T	:	:	:
W	:	:	:
T	:	:	:
F	:	:	:
S	:	:	:
S	:	:	:

	START TIME	END TIME	TOTAL FAST HRS
M	:	:	:
T	:	:	:
W	:	:	:
T	:	:	:
F	:	:	:
S	:	:	:
S	:	:	:

	START TIME	END TIME	TOTAL FAST HRS
M	:	:	:
T	:	:	:
W	:	:	:
T	:	:	:
F	:	:	:
S	:	:	:
S	:	:	:

	START TIME	END TIME	TOTAL FAST HRS
M	:	:	:
T	:	:	:
W	:	:	:
T	:	:	:
F	:	:	:
S	:	:	:
S	:	:	:

NOTES & REFLECTIONS

MILESTONES & ACCOMPLISHMENTS

GOALS &
Accomplishments

MONTH | JAN FEB MAR APR MAY JUN JUL AUG SEP OCT NOV DEC

THIS MONTH'S GOALS

ACTION PLAN

	M	T	W	T	F	S	S
	☐	☐	☐	☐	☐	☐	☐
	☐	☐	☐	☐	☐	☐	☐
	☐	☐	☐	☐	☐	☐	☐
	☐	☐	☐	☐	☐	☐	☐
	☐	☐	☐	☐	☐	☐	☐

NOTES:

WEEKLY GOALS

THOUGHTS

MEAL IDEAS:	BREAKFAST	LUNCH	DINNER	SNACKS
M				
T				
W				
T				
F				
S				
S				

MY DAILY PROGRESS **Tracker**

SLEEP TRACKER:

DATE _____

☼ RISE: _____   🌙 zᶻᶻ BEDTIME: _____   💤 SLEEP (HRS): _____

NOTES FOR THE DAY

_____

_____

_____

FASTING TIMES & DURATION

EXERCISE / WORKOUT ROUTINE

TOP 6 PRIORITIES OF THE DAY

- ⦿ _____   ⦿ _____
- ⦿ _____   ⦿ _____
- ⦿ _____   ⦿ _____

IN A STATE OF KETOSIS?

YES   NO   UNSURE

WATER INTAKE TRACKER

DAILY ENERGY LEVEL		
HIGH	**MEDIUM**	**LOW**

1ˢᵗ MEAL

FAT: CARBS: PROTEIN: CALORIES:

2ⁿᵈ MEAL

FAT: CARBS: PROTEIN: CALORIES:

Other MEALS & SNACKS

FAT: CARBS: PROTEIN: CALORIES:

END OF THE DAY TOTAL OVERVIEW

FAT   CARBS   PROTEIN   KCAL

MY DAILY PROGRESS **Tracker**

SLEEP TRACKER:

DATE

RISE:

BEDTIME:

SLEEP (HRS):

NOTES FOR THE DAY

IN A STATE OF KETOSIS?

YES   NO   UNSURE

WATER INTAKE TRACKER

FASTING TIMES & DURATION

DAILY ENERGY LEVEL

HIGH   **MEDIUM**   **LOW**

1st MEAL

FAT: CARBS: PROTEIN: CALORIES:

EXERCISE / WORKOUT ROUTINE

2nd MEAL

FAT: CARBS: PROTEIN: CALORIES:

Other MEALS & SNACKS

FAT: CARBS: PROTEIN: CALORIES:

TOP 6 PRIORITIES OF THE DAY

END OF THE DAY TOTAL OVERVIEW

FAT   CARBS   PROTEIN   KCAL

MY DAILY PROGRESS **Tracker**

DATE _____

SLEEP TRACKER:

RISE: _____   BEDTIME: _____   SLEEP (HRS): _____

NOTES FOR THE DAY

_____

_____

_____

FASTING TIMES & DURATION

EXERCISE / WORKOUT ROUTINE

TOP 6 PRIORITIES OF THE DAY

- ○ _____   ○ _____
- ○ _____   ○ _____
- ○ _____   ○ _____

IN A STATE OF KETOSIS?

YES   NO   UNSURE

WATER INTAKE TRACKER

DAILY ENERGY LEVEL		
HIGH	**MEDIUM**	**LOW**

1st MEAL

FAT: CARBS: PROTEIN: CALORIES:

2nd MEAL

FAT: CARBS: PROTEIN: CALORIES:

Other MEALS & SNACKS

FAT: CARBS: PROTEIN: CALORIES:

END OF THE DAY TOTAL OVERVIEW

FAT	CARBS	PROTEIN	KCAL

MY DAILY PROGRESS **Tracker**

SLEEP TRACKER:

DATE _____

RISE: _____   BEDTIME: _____   SLEEP (HRS): _____

NOTES FOR THE DAY

_____
_____
_____

IN A STATE OF KETOSIS?

YES   NO   UNSURE

WATER INTAKE TRACKER

FASTING TIMES & DURATION

DAILY ENERGY LEVEL

HIGH	MEDIUM	LOW

1st MEAL

FAT: CARBS: PROTEIN: CALORIES:

EXERCISE / WORKOUT ROUTINE

2nd MEAL

FAT: CARBS: PROTEIN: CALORIES:

Other MEALS & SNACKS

FAT: CARBS: PROTEIN: CALORIES:

TOP 6 PRIORITIES OF THE DAY

END OF THE DAY TOTAL OVERVIEW

FAT   CARBS   PROTEIN   KCAL

MY DAILY PROGRESS **Tracker**

SLEEP TRACKER:

DATE

RISE:

BEDTIME:

SLEEP (HRS):

NOTES FOR THE DAY

IN A STATE OF KETOSIS?

YES   NO   UNSURE

WATER INTAKE TRACKER

FASTING TIMES & DURATION

DAILY ENERGY LEVEL		
HIGH	**MEDIUM**	**LOW**

1st MEAL

FAT: CARBS: PROTEIN: CALORIES:

EXERCISE / WORKOUT ROUTINE

2nd MEAL

FAT: CARBS: PROTEIN: CALORIES:

Other MEALS & SNACKS

FAT: CARBS: PROTEIN: CALORIES:

TOP 6 PRIORITIES OF THE DAY

END OF THE DAY TOTAL OVERVIEW

FAT   CARBS   PROTEIN   KCAL

MEAL Planner

GROCERY LIST

MON

TUES

WED

THUR

FRI

SAT

SUN

My SHOPPING LIST

FRESH PRODUCE

MEAT AND SEAFOOD

DAIRY PRODUCTS

PANTRY ITEMS

FROZEN / OTHER

MY DAILY PROGRESS **Tracker**

SLEEP TRACKER:

DATE _____

| ☀ | RISE: | 🌙 zᶻᶻ | BEDTIME: | 💭 z+z | SLEEP (HRS): |

NOTES FOR THE DAY

_____

_____

_____

FASTING TIMES & DURATION

EXERCISE / WORKOUT ROUTINE

TOP 6 PRIORITIES OF THE DAY

- _____ ○ _____
- _____ ○ _____
- _____ ○ _____

IN A STATE OF KETOSIS?

YES   NO   UNSURE

WATER INTAKE TRACKER

DAILY ENERGY LEVEL

| **HIGH** | **MEDIUM** | **LOW** |

1ˢᵗ MEAL

FAT: CARBS: PROTEIN: CALORIES:

2ⁿᵈ MEAL

FAT: CARBS: PROTEIN: CALORIES:

Other MEALS & SNACKS

FAT: CARBS: PROTEIN: CALORIES:

END OF THE DAY TOTAL OVERVIEW

FAT   CARBS   PROTEIN   KCAL

MY DAILY PROGRESS **Tracker**

SLEEP TRACKER:

DATE _____

RISE: _____

BEDTIME: _____

SLEEP (HRS): _____

NOTES FOR THE DAY

_____

_____

_____

FASTING TIMES & DURATION

EXERCISE / WORKOUT ROUTINE

TOP 6 PRIORITIES OF THE DAY

- _____ _____
- _____ _____
- _____ _____

IN A STATE OF KETOSIS?

YES   NO   UNSURE

WATER INTAKE TRACKER

DAILY ENERGY LEVEL		
HIGH	**MEDIUM**	**LOW**

1st MEAL

FAT: CARBS: PROTEIN: CALORIES:

2nd MEAL

FAT: CARBS: PROTEIN: CALORIES:

Other MEALS & SNACKS

FAT: CARBS: PROTEIN: CALORIES:

END OF THE DAY TOTAL OVERVIEW

FAT	CARBS	PROTEIN	KCAL

MY DAILY PROGRESS **Tracker**

SLEEP TRACKER:

DATE _____

RISE: _____   BEDTIME: _____   SLEEP (HRS): _____

NOTES FOR THE DAY

_____
_____
_____

FASTING TIMES & DURATION

EXERCISE / WORKOUT ROUTINE

TOP 6 PRIORITIES OF THE DAY

_____   _____
_____   _____
_____   _____

IN A STATE OF KETOSIS?

YES   NO   UNSURE

WATER INTAKE TRACKER

DAILY ENERGY LEVEL

HIGH   **MEDIUM**   **LOW**

1st MEAL

FAT: CARBS: PROTEIN: CALORIES:

2nd MEAL

FAT: CARBS: PROTEIN: CALORIES:

Other MEALS & SNACKS

FAT: CARBS: PROTEIN: CALORIES:

END OF THE DAY TOTAL OVERVIEW

FAT   CARBS   PROTEIN   KCAL

MY DAILY PROGRESS **Tracker**

SLEEP TRACKER:

DATE

RISE: BEDTIME: SLEEP (HRS):

NOTES FOR THE DAY

IN A STATE OF KETOSIS?

YES   NO   UNSURE

WATER INTAKE TRACKER

FASTING TIMES & DURATION

DAILY ENERGY LEVEL		
HIGH	**MEDIUM**	**LOW**

1st MEAL

FAT: CARBS: PROTEIN: CALORIES:

2nd MEAL

FAT: CARBS: PROTEIN: CALORIES:

Other MEALS & SNACKS

FAT: CARBS: PROTEIN: CALORIES:

EXERCISE / WORKOUT ROUTINE

TOP 6 PRIORITIES OF THE DAY

END OF THE DAY TOTAL OVERVIEW

FAT   CARBS   PROTEIN   KCAL

MY DAILY PROGRESS **Tracker**

SLEEP TRACKER:

DATE _____

RISE: _____

BEDTIME: _____

SLEEP (HRS): _____

NOTES FOR THE DAY

_____
_____
_____
_____

FASTING TIMES & DURATION

EXERCISE / WORKOUT ROUTINE

TOP 6 PRIORITIES OF THE DAY

- ○ _____ ○ _____
- ○ _____ ○ _____
- ○ _____ ○ _____

IN A STATE OF KETOSIS?

YES   NO   UNSURE

WATER INTAKE TRACKER

DAILY ENERGY LEVEL

HIGH	**MEDIUM**	**LOW**

1st MEAL

FAT: CARBS: PROTEIN: CALORIES:

2nd MEAL

FAT: CARBS: PROTEIN: CALORIES:

Other MEALS & SNACKS

FAT: CARBS: PROTEIN: CALORIES:

END OF THE DAY TOTAL OVERVIEW

FAT	CARBS	PROTEIN	KCAL

MY DAILY PROGRESS **Tracker**

SLEEP TRACKER:

DATE _____

RISE: _____

BEDTIME: _____

SLEEP (HRS): _____

NOTES FOR THE DAY

_____

_____

_____

IN A STATE OF KETOSIS?

YES   NO   UNSURE

WATER INTAKE TRACKER

FASTING TIMES & DURATION

DAILY ENERGY LEVEL

HIGH	**MEDIUM**	**LOW**

1st MEAL

FAT: CARBS: PROTEIN: CALORIES:

EXERCISE / WORKOUT ROUTINE

2nd MEAL

FAT: CARBS: PROTEIN: CALORIES:

Other MEALS & SNACKS

FAT: CARBS: PROTEIN: CALORIES:

TOP 6 PRIORITIES OF THE DAY

END OF THE DAY TOTAL OVERVIEW

FAT	CARBS	PROTEIN	KCAL

MY DAILY PROGRESS **Tracker**

SLEEP TRACKER:

DATE _____

RISE: _____

BEDTIME: _____

SLEEP (HRS): _____

NOTES FOR THE DAY

_____
_____
_____

IN A STATE OF KETOSIS?

YES   NO   UNSURE

WATER INTAKE TRACKER

FASTING TIMES & DURATION

DAILY ENERGY LEVEL

HIGH   **MEDIUM**   **LOW**

1st MEAL

FAT: CARBS: PROTEIN: CALORIES:

EXERCISE / WORKOUT ROUTINE

2nd MEAL

FAT: CARBS: PROTEIN: CALORIES:

Other MEALS & SNACKS

FAT: CARBS: PROTEIN: CALORIES:

TOP 6 PRIORITIES OF THE DAY

END OF THE DAY TOTAL OVERVIEW

FAT   CARBS   PROTEIN   KCAL

MEAL **Planner**

WEEK OF

GROCERY LIST

- [ ]
- [ ]
- [ ]
- [ ]
- [ ]
- [ ]
- [ ]
- [ ]
- [ ]
- [ ]
- [ ]
- [ ]
- [ ]
- [ ]
- [ ]
- [ ]

MON

TUES

WED

THUR

FRI

SAT

SUN

My SHOPPING LIST

FRESH PRODUCE

MEAT AND SEAFOOD

DAIRY PRODUCTS

PANTRY ITEMS

FROZEN / OTHER

MY DAILY PROGRESS **Tracker**

SLEEP TRACKER:

DATE _____

☼ RISE: _____

🌙 z z z BEDTIME: _____

💤 SLEEP (HRS): _____

NOTES FOR THE DAY

_____

_____

_____

FASTING TIMES & DURATION

EXERCISE / WORKOUT ROUTINE

TOP 6 PRIORITIES OF THE DAY

○ _____   ○ _____

○ _____   ○ _____

○ _____   ○ _____

IN A STATE OF KETOSIS?

YES   NO   UNSURE

WATER INTAKE TRACKER

💧 💧 💧 💧 💧 💧 💧 💧

DAILY ENERGY LEVEL		
HIGH	**MEDIUM**	**LOW**

1st MEAL

FAT: CARBS: PROTEIN: CALORIES:

2nd MEAL

FAT: CARBS: PROTEIN: CALORIES:

Other MEALS & SNACKS

FAT: CARBS: PROTEIN: CALORIES:

END OF THE DAY TOTAL OVERVIEW

FAT   CARBS   PROTEIN   KCAL

MY DAILY PROGRESS **Tracker**

SLEEP TRACKER:

DATE _____

RISE: _____   BEDTIME: _____   SLEEP (HRS): _____

NOTES FOR THE DAY

_____

_____

_____

IN A STATE OF KETOSIS?

YES   NO   UNSURE

WATER INTAKE TRACKER

FASTING TIMES & DURATION

DAILY ENERGY LEVEL

HIGH   **MEDIUM**   **LOW**

1st MEAL

FAT: CARBS: PROTEIN: CALORIES:

2nd MEAL

FAT: CARBS: PROTEIN: CALORIES:

Other MEALS & SNACKS

FAT: CARBS: PROTEIN: CALORIES:

EXERCISE / WORKOUT ROUTINE

TOP 6 PRIORITIES OF THE DAY

END OF THE DAY TOTAL OVERVIEW

FAT   CARBS   PROTEIN   KCAL

MY DAILY PROGRESS **Tracker**

SLEEP TRACKER:

DATE _____

RISE: _____   BEDTIME: _____   SLEEP (HRS): _____

NOTES FOR THE DAY

_____

_____

_____

IN A STATE OF KETOSIS?

YES   NO   UNSURE

WATER INTAKE TRACKER

FASTING TIMES & DURATION

DAILY ENERGY LEVEL

HIGH	MEDIUM	LOW

1st MEAL

FAT: CARBS: PROTEIN: CALORIES:

EXERCISE / WORKOUT ROUTINE

2nd MEAL

FAT: CARBS: PROTEIN: CALORIES:

Other MEALS & SNACKS

FAT: CARBS: PROTEIN: CALORIES:

TOP 6 PRIORITIES OF THE DAY

END OF THE DAY TOTAL OVERVIEW

FAT   CARBS   PROTEIN   KCAL

MY DAILY PROGRESS **Tracker**

SLEEP TRACKER:

DATE _____

RISE: _____   BEDTIME: _____   SLEEP (HRS): _____

NOTES FOR THE DAY

_____

_____

_____

IN A STATE OF KETOSIS?

YES   NO   UNSURE

WATER INTAKE TRACKER

FASTING TIMES & DURATION

DAILY ENERGY LEVEL		
HIGH	**MEDIUM**	**LOW**

1st MEAL

FAT: CARBS: PROTEIN: CALORIES:

EXERCISE / WORKOUT ROUTINE

2nd MEAL

FAT: CARBS: PROTEIN: CALORIES:

Other MEALS & SNACKS

FAT: CARBS: PROTEIN: CALORIES:

TOP 6 PRIORITIES OF THE DAY

END OF THE DAY TOTAL OVERVIEW

FAT   CARBS   PROTEIN   KCAL

MY DAILY PROGRESS **Tracker**

SLEEP TRACKER:

DATE _____

RISE: _____   BEDTIME: _____   SLEEP (HRS): _____

NOTES FOR THE DAY

_____

_____

_____

FASTING TIMES & DURATION

EXERCISE / WORKOUT ROUTINE

TOP 6 PRIORITIES OF THE DAY

○ _____   ○ _____

○ _____   ○ _____

○ _____   ○ _____

IN A STATE OF KETOSIS?

YES   NO   UNSURE

WATER INTAKE TRACKER

DAILY ENERGY LEVEL

HIGH   **MEDIUM**   **LOW**

1st MEAL

FAT: CARBS: PROTEIN: CALORIES:

2nd MEAL

FAT: CARBS: PROTEIN: CALORIES:

Other MEALS & SNACKS

FAT: CARBS: PROTEIN: CALORIES:

END OF THE DAY TOTAL OVERVIEW

FAT   CARBS   PROTEIN   KCAL

_____   _____   _____   _____

MY DAILY PROGRESS **Tracker**

SLEEP TRACKER:

DATE _____

☀ RISE: [_____]   🌙 BEDTIME: [_____]   💤 SLEEP (HRS): [_____]

NOTES FOR THE DAY

_____
_____
_____

FASTING TIMES & DURATION

EXERCISE / WORKOUT ROUTINE

TOP 6 PRIORITIES OF THE DAY

○ _____   ○ _____
○ _____   ○ _____
○ _____   ○ _____

IN A STATE OF KETOSIS?

YES   NO   UNSURE

WATER INTAKE TRACKER

DAILY ENERGY LEVEL		
HIGH	**MEDIUM**	**LOW**

1st MEAL

FAT: CARBS: PROTEIN: CALORIES:

2nd MEAL

FAT: CARBS: PROTEIN: CALORIES:

Other MEALS & SNACKS

FAT: CARBS: PROTEIN: CALORIES:

END OF THE DAY TOTAL OVERVIEW

FAT	CARBS	PROTEIN	KCAL

MY DAILY PROGRESS **Tracker**

SLEEP TRACKER:

DATE

RISE:

BEDTIME:

SLEEP (HRS):

NOTES FOR THE DAY

IN A STATE OF KETOSIS?

YES   NO   UNSURE

WATER INTAKE TRACKER

FASTING TIMES & DURATION

DAILY ENERGY LEVEL		
HIGH	**MEDIUM**	**LOW**

1st MEAL

FAT: CARBS: PROTEIN: CALORIES:

EXERCISE / WORKOUT ROUTINE

2nd MEAL

FAT: CARBS: PROTEIN: CALORIES:

Other MEALS & SNACKS

FAT: CARBS: PROTEIN: CALORIES:

TOP 6 PRIORITIES OF THE DAY

END OF THE DAY TOTAL OVERVIEW

FAT   CARBS   PROTEIN   KCAL

MEAL Planner

GROCERY LIST

- ☐
- ☐
- ☐
- ☐
- ☐
- ☐
- ☐
- ☐
- ☐
- ☐
- ☐
- ☐
- ☐
- ☐
- ☐
- ☐
- ☐
- ☐

MON

TUES

WED

THUR

FRI

SAT

SUN

My SHOPPING LIST

FRESH PRODUCE

MEAT AND SEAFOOD

DAIRY PRODUCTS

PANTRY ITEMS

FROZEN / OTHER

MY DAILY PROGRESS **Tracker**

SLEEP TRACKER:

DATE _____

RISE: _____   BEDTIME: _____   SLEEP (HRS): _____

NOTES FOR THE DAY

_____

_____

_____

FASTING TIMES & DURATION

EXERCISE / WORKOUT ROUTINE

TOP 6 PRIORITIES OF THE DAY

IN A STATE OF KETOSIS?

YES   NO   UNSURE

WATER INTAKE TRACKER

DAILY ENERGY LEVEL		
HIGH	**MEDIUM**	**LOW**

1st MEAL

FAT: CARBS: PROTEIN: CALORIES:

2nd MEAL

FAT: CARBS: PROTEIN: CALORIES:

Other MEALS & SNACKS

FAT: CARBS: PROTEIN: CALORIES:

END OF THE DAY TOTAL OVERVIEW

FAT   CARBS   PROTEIN   KCAL

MY DAILY PROGRESS **Tracker**

SLEEP TRACKER:

DATE _____

RISE: _____   BEDTIME: _____   SLEEP (HRS): _____

NOTES FOR THE DAY

_____
_____
_____

FASTING TIMES & DURATION

EXERCISE / WORKOUT ROUTINE

TOP 6 PRIORITIES OF THE DAY

_____   _____
_____   _____
_____   _____

IN A STATE OF KETOSIS?

YES   NO   UNSURE

WATER INTAKE TRACKER

DAILY ENERGY LEVEL

HIGH	MEDIUM	LOW

1st MEAL

FAT: CARBS: PROTEIN: CALORIES:

2nd MEAL

FAT: CARBS: PROTEIN: CALORIES:

Other MEALS & SNACKS

FAT: CARBS: PROTEIN: CALORIES:

END OF THE DAY TOTAL OVERVIEW

FAT	CARBS	PROTEIN	KCAL

MY DAILY PROGRESS **Tracker**

SLEEP TRACKER:

DATE _____

☀ RISE: _____   🌙 BEDTIME: _____   💤 SLEEP (HRS): _____

NOTES FOR THE DAY

_____
_____
_____

IN A STATE OF KETOSIS?

YES   NO   UNSURE

WATER INTAKE TRACKER

FASTING TIMES & DURATION

DAILY ENERGY LEVEL

HIGH   **MEDIUM**   **LOW**

1st MEAL

FAT: CARBS: PROTEIN: CALORIES:

EXERCISE / WORKOUT ROUTINE

2nd MEAL

FAT: CARBS: PROTEIN: CALORIES:

Other MEALS & SNACKS

FAT: CARBS: PROTEIN: CALORIES:

TOP 6 PRIORITIES OF THE DAY

END OF THE DAY TOTAL OVERVIEW

FAT   CARBS   PROTEIN   KCAL

MY DAILY PROGRESS **Tracker**

SLEEP TRACKER:

DATE

RISE:　　　　BEDTIME:　　　　SLEEP (HRS):

NOTES FOR THE DAY

IN A STATE OF KETOSIS?

YES　　　NO　　　UNSURE

WATER INTAKE TRACKER

FASTING TIMES & DURATION

DAILY ENERGY LEVEL

HIGH	MEDIUM	LOW

1st MEAL

FAT:　　CARBS:　　PROTEIN:　　CALORIES:

2nd MEAL

FAT:　　CARBS:　　PROTEIN:　　CALORIES:

EXERCISE / WORKOUT ROUTINE

Other MEALS & SNACKS

FAT:　　CARBS:　　PROTEIN:　　CALORIES:

TOP 6 PRIORITIES OF THE DAY

END OF THE DAY TOTAL OVERVIEW

FAT　　　CARBS　　　PROTEIN　　　KCAL

MY DAILY PROGRESS **Tracker**

SLEEP TRACKER:

DATE _____

RISE: _____

BEDTIME: _____

SLEEP (HRS): _____

NOTES FOR THE DAY

_____

_____

IN A STATE OF KETOSIS?

YES   NO   UNSURE

WATER INTAKE TRACKER

FASTING TIMES & DURATION

EXERCISE / WORKOUT ROUTINE

TOP 6 PRIORITIES OF THE DAY

DAILY ENERGY LEVEL

HIGH   **MEDIUM**   **LOW**

1st MEAL

FAT: CARBS: PROTEIN: CALORIES:

2nd MEAL

FAT: CARBS: PROTEIN: CALORIES:

Other MEALS & SNACKS

FAT: CARBS: PROTEIN: CALORIES:

END OF THE DAY TOTAL OVERVIEW

FAT   CARBS   PROTEIN   KCAL

MY DAILY PROGRESS Tracker

SLEEP TRACKER:

DATE _____

☀ RISE: _____   🌙 z_z^z BEDTIME: _____   💤 SLEEP (HRS): _____

NOTES FOR THE DAY

_____
_____
_____

FASTING TIMES & DURATION

EXERCISE / WORKOUT ROUTINE

TOP 6 PRIORITIES OF THE DAY

○ _____   ○ _____
○ _____   ○ _____
○ _____   ○ _____

IN A STATE OF KETOSIS?

YES   NO   UNSURE

WATER INTAKE TRACKER

DAILY ENERGY LEVEL

HIGH   **MEDIUM**   **LOW**

1st MEAL

FAT: CARBS: PROTEIN: CALORIES:

2nd MEAL

FAT: CARBS: PROTEIN: CALORIES:

Other MEALS & SNACKS

FAT: CARBS: PROTEIN: CALORIES:

END OF THE DAY TOTAL OVERVIEW

FAT   CARBS   PROTEIN   KCAL

MY DAILY PROGRESS **Tracker**

SLEEP TRACKER:

DATE

RISE:

BEDTIME:

SLEEP (HRS):

NOTES FOR THE DAY

IN A STATE OF KETOSIS?

YES   NO   UNSURE

WATER INTAKE TRACKER

FASTING TIMES & DURATION

DAILY ENERGY LEVEL		
HIGH	**MEDIUM**	**LOW**

1st MEAL

FAT: CARBS: PROTEIN: CALORIES:

EXERCISE / WORKOUT ROUTINE

2nd MEAL

FAT: CARBS: PROTEIN: CALORIES:

Other MEALS & SNACKS

FAT: CARBS: PROTEIN: CALORIES:

TOP 6 PRIORITIES OF THE DAY

END OF THE DAY TOTAL OVERVIEW

FAT   CARBS   PROTEIN   KCAL

MEAL **Planner**

WEEK OF

GROCERY LIST

- [ ]
- [ ]
- [ ]
- [ ]
- [ ]
- [ ]
- [ ]
- [ ]
- [ ]
- [ ]
- [ ]
- [ ]
- [ ]
- [ ]
- [ ]
- [ ]
- [ ]
- [ ]
- [ ]

MON

TUES

WED

THUR

FRI

SAT

SUN

My SHOPPING LIST

FRESH PRODUCE

MEAT AND SEAFOOD

DAIRY PRODUCTS

PANTRY ITEMS

FROZEN / OTHER

MY DAILY PROGRESS **Tracker**

SLEEP TRACKER:

DATE _____

RISE: _____   BEDTIME: _____   SLEEP (HRS): _____

NOTES FOR THE DAY

_____
_____
_____

IN A STATE OF KETOSIS?

YES   NO   UNSURE

WATER INTAKE TRACKER

FASTING TIMES & DURATION

DAILY ENERGY LEVEL

HIGH	**MEDIUM**	**LOW**

1st MEAL

FAT: CARBS: PROTEIN: CALORIES:

2nd MEAL

FAT: CARBS: PROTEIN: CALORIES:

Other MEALS & SNACKS

FAT: CARBS: PROTEIN: CALORIES:

EXERCISE / WORKOUT ROUTINE

TOP 6 PRIORITIES OF THE DAY

END OF THE DAY TOTAL OVERVIEW

FAT   CARBS   PROTEIN   KCAL

MY DAILY PROGRESS **Tracker**

SLEEP TRACKER:

DATE _____

RISE: _____

BEDTIME: _____

SLEEP (HRS): _____

NOTES FOR THE DAY

_____
_____
_____

IN A STATE OF KETOSIS?

YES   NO   UNSURE

WATER INTAKE TRACKER

FASTING TIMES & DURATION

DAILY ENERGY LEVEL

HIGH   **MEDIUM**   **LOW**

1st MEAL

FAT: CARBS: PROTEIN: CALORIES:

2nd MEAL

FAT: CARBS: PROTEIN: CALORIES:

Other MEALS & SNACKS

FAT: CARBS: PROTEIN: CALORIES:

EXERCISE / WORKOUT ROUTINE

TOP 6 PRIORITIES OF THE DAY

END OF THE DAY TOTAL OVERVIEW

FAT   CARBS   PROTEIN   KCAL

MY DAILY PROGRESS **Tracker**

SLEEP TRACKER:

DATE _____

RISE: _____   BEDTIME: _____   SLEEP (HRS): _____

NOTES FOR THE DAY

_____

_____

_____

IN A STATE OF KETOSIS?

YES   NO   UNSURE

WATER INTAKE TRACKER

FASTING TIMES & DURATION

DAILY ENERGY LEVEL

HIGH	**MEDIUM**	**LOW**

1ˢᵗ MEAL

FAT: CARBS: PROTEIN: CALORIES:

2ⁿᵈ MEAL

FAT: CARBS: PROTEIN: CALORIES:

EXERCISE / WORKOUT ROUTINE

Other MEALS & SNACKS

FAT: CARBS: PROTEIN: CALORIES:

TOP 6 PRIORITIES OF THE DAY

END OF THE DAY TOTAL OVERVIEW

FAT   CARBS   PROTEIN   KCAL

MY DAILY PROGRESS **Tracker**

SLEEP TRACKER:

DATE _____

RISE: _____   BEDTIME: _____   SLEEP (HRS): _____

NOTES FOR THE DAY

_____

_____

_____

FASTING TIMES & DURATION

EXERCISE / WORKOUT ROUTINE

TOP 6 PRIORITIES OF THE DAY

IN A STATE OF KETOSIS?

YES   NO   UNSURE

WATER INTAKE TRACKER

DAILY ENERGY LEVEL		
HIGH	**MEDIUM**	**LOW**

1st MEAL

FAT: CARBS: PROTEIN: CALORIES:

2nd MEAL

FAT: CARBS: PROTEIN: CALORIES:

Other MEALS & SNACKS

FAT: CARBS: PROTEIN: CALORIES:

END OF THE DAY TOTAL OVERVIEW

FAT   CARBS   PROTEIN   KCAL

WEIGHT LOSS **Tracker**

WEEKLY WEIGHT LOSS TRACKER

MONTHLY GOAL

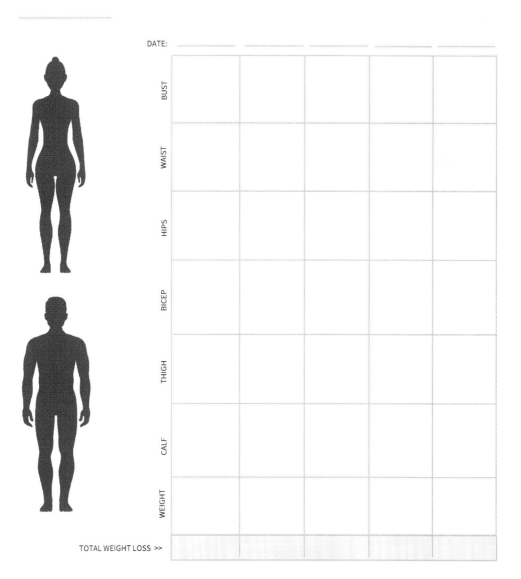

DATE:

	BUST				
	WAIST				
	HIPS				
	BICEP				
	THIGH				
	CALF				
	WEIGHT				

TOTAL WEIGHT LOSS >>

INTERMITTENT Fasting Log

WEEK OF:

	START TIME	END TIME	TOTAL FAST HRS
M	:	:	:
T	:	:	:
W	:	:	:
T	:	:	:
F	:	:	:
S	:	:	:
S	:	:	:

WEEK OF:

	START TIME	END TIME	TOTAL FAST HRS
M	:	:	:
T	:	:	:
W	:	:	:
T	:	:	:
F	:	:	:
S	:	:	:
S	:	:	:

WEEK OF:

	START TIME	END TIME	TOTAL FAST HRS
M	:	:	:
T	:	:	:
W	:	:	:
T	:	:	:
F	:	:	:
S	:	:	:
S	:	:	:

WEEK OF:

	START TIME	END TIME	TOTAL FAST HRS
M	:	:	:
T	:	:	:
W	:	:	:
T	:	:	:
F	:	:	:
S	:	:	:
S	:	:	:

WEEK OF:

	START TIME	END TIME	TOTAL FAST HRS
M	:	:	:
T	:	:	:
W	:	:	:
T	:	:	:
F	:	:	:
S	:	:	:
S	:	:	:

NOTES & REFLECTIONS

MILESTONES & ACCOMPLISHMENTS

GOALS &
Accomplishments

Month | JAN FEB MAR APR MAY JUN JUL AUG SEP OCT NOV DEC

THIS MONTH'S GOALS

ACTION PLAN

M T W T F S S

☐☐☐☐☐☐☐
☐☐☐☐☐☐☐
☐☐☐☐☐☐☐
☐☐☐☐☐☐☐
☐☐☐☐☐☐☐

NOTES:

WEEKLY GOALS

THOUGHTS

MEAL IDEAS:	BREAKFAST	LUNCH	DINNER	SNACKS
M				
T				
W				
T				
F				
S				
S				

MY DAILY PROGRESS **Tracker**

SLEEP TRACKER:

DATE _____

RISE: _____   BEDTIME: _____   SLEEP (HRS): _____

NOTES FOR THE DAY

_____

_____

_____

FASTING TIMES & DURATION

EXERCISE / WORKOUT ROUTINE

TOP 6 PRIORITIES OF THE DAY

IN A STATE OF KETOSIS?

YES   NO   UNSURE

WATER INTAKE TRACKER

DAILY ENERGY LEVEL

HIGH   **MEDIUM**   **LOW**

1st MEAL

FAT: CARBS: PROTEIN: CALORIES:

2nd MEAL

FAT: CARBS: PROTEIN: CALORIES:

Other MEALS & SNACKS

FAT: CARBS: PROTEIN: CALORIES:

END OF THE DAY TOTAL OVERVIEW

FAT   CARBS   PROTEIN   KCAL

MY DAILY PROGRESS **Tracker**

SLEEP TRACKER:

DATE _____

RISE: _____ BEDTIME: _____ SLEEP (HRS): _____

NOTES FOR THE DAY

_____

_____

_____

FASTING TIMES & DURATION

EXERCISE / WORKOUT ROUTINE

TOP 6 PRIORITIES OF THE DAY

IN A STATE OF KETOSIS?

YES   NO   UNSURE

WATER INTAKE TRACKER

DAILY ENERGY LEVEL		
HIGH	**MEDIUM**	**LOW**

1st MEAL

FAT: CARBS: PROTEIN: CALORIES:

2nd MEAL

FAT: CARBS: PROTEIN: CALORIES:

Other MEALS & SNACKS

FAT: CARBS: PROTEIN: CALORIES:

END OF THE DAY TOTAL OVERVIEW

FAT   CARBS   PROTEIN   KCAL

MY DAILY PROGRESS **Tracker**

SLEEP TRACKER:

DATE _____

☀ RISE: _____   🌙 z z z BEDTIME: _____   💤 SLEEP (HRS): _____

NOTES FOR THE DAY

_____

_____

_____

FASTING TIMES & DURATION

EXERCISE / WORKOUT ROUTINE

TOP 6 PRIORITIES OF THE DAY

IN A STATE OF KETOSIS?

YES   NO   UNSURE

WATER INTAKE TRACKER

DAILY ENERGY LEVEL		
HIGH	**MEDIUM**	**LOW**

1st MEAL

FAT: CARBS: PROTEIN: CALORIES:

2nd MEAL

FAT: CARBS: PROTEIN: CALORIES:

Other MEALS & SNACKS

FAT: CARBS: PROTEIN: CALORIES:

END OF THE DAY TOTAL OVERVIEW

FAT   CARBS   PROTEIN   KCAL

_____   _____   _____   _____

MEAL **Planner**

WEEK OF

GROCERY LIST

- ☐
- ☐
- ☐
- ☐
- ☐
- ☐
- ☐
- ☐
- ☐
- ☐
- ☐
- ☐
- ☐
- ☐
- ☐
- ☐
- ☐
- ☐
- ☐

MON

TUES

WED

THUR

FRI

SAT

SUN

My SHOPPING LIST

FRESH PRODUCE

MEAT AND SEAFOOD

DAIRY PRODUCTS

PANTRY ITEMS

FROZEN / OTHER

MY DAILY PROGRESS **Tracker**

SLEEP TRACKER:

DATE _____

| RISE: | BEDTIME: | SLEEP (HRS): |

NOTES FOR THE DAY

_____
_____
_____

IN A STATE OF KETOSIS?

YES   NO   UNSURE

WATER INTAKE TRACKER

FASTING TIMES & DURATION

DAILY ENERGY LEVEL

| **HIGH** | **MEDIUM** | **LOW** |

1st MEAL

FAT: CARBS: PROTEIN: CALORIES:

2nd MEAL

FAT: CARBS: PROTEIN: CALORIES:

EXERCISE / WORKOUT ROUTINE

Other MEALS & SNACKS

FAT: CARBS: PROTEIN: CALORIES:

TOP 6 PRIORITIES OF THE DAY

END OF THE DAY TOTAL OVERVIEW

| FAT | CARBS | PROTEIN | KCAL |

MY DAILY PROGRESS **Tracker**

SLEEP TRACKER:

DATE _____

RISE: _____ BEDTIME: _____ SLEEP (HRS): _____

NOTES FOR THE DAY
_____
_____
_____

IN A STATE OF KETOSIS?

YES   NO   UNSURE

WATER INTAKE TRACKER

FASTING TIMES & DURATION

EXERCISE / WORKOUT ROUTINE

DAILY ENERGY LEVEL

HIGH   **MEDIUM**   **LOW**

1st MEAL

FAT: CARBS: PROTEIN: CALORIES:

2nd MEAL

FAT: CARBS: PROTEIN: CALORIES:

Other MEALS & SNACKS

FAT: CARBS: PROTEIN: CALORIES:

TOP 6 PRIORITIES OF THE DAY

END OF THE DAY TOTAL OVERVIEW

FAT   CARBS   PROTEIN   KCAL

MY DAILY PROGRESS **Tracker**

SLEEP TRACKER:

DATE _____

RISE: _____   BEDTIME: _____   SLEEP (HRS): _____

NOTES FOR THE DAY

_____
_____
_____

FASTING TIMES & DURATION

EXERCISE / WORKOUT ROUTINE

TOP 6 PRIORITIES OF THE DAY

IN A STATE OF KETOSIS?

YES   NO   UNSURE

WATER INTAKE TRACKER

DAILY ENERGY LEVEL

HIGH   **MEDIUM**   **LOW**

1st MEAL

FAT: CARBS: PROTEIN: CALORIES:

2nd MEAL

FAT: CARBS: PROTEIN: CALORIES:

Other MEALS & SNACKS

FAT: CARBS: PROTEIN: CALORIES:

END OF THE DAY TOTAL OVERVIEW

FAT   CARBS   PROTEIN   KCAL

MY DAILY PROGRESS **Tracker**

SLEEP TRACKER:

DATE _____

RISE: _____   BEDTIME: _____   SLEEP (HRS): _____

NOTES FOR THE DAY

_____

_____

_____

IN A STATE OF KETOSIS?

YES   NO   UNSURE

WATER INTAKE TRACKER

FASTING TIMES & DURATION

DAILY ENERGY LEVEL

HIGH   **MEDIUM**   **LOW**

1st **MEAL**

FAT: CARBS: PROTEIN: CALORIES:

EXERCISE / WORKOUT ROUTINE

2nd **MEAL**

FAT: CARBS: PROTEIN: CALORIES:

Other **MEALS & SNACKS**

FAT: CARBS: PROTEIN: CALORIES:

TOP 6 PRIORITIES OF THE DAY

END OF THE DAY TOTAL OVERVIEW

FAT   CARBS   PROTEIN   KCAL

MY DAILY PROGRESS **Tracker**

SLEEP TRACKER:

DATE _____

RISE: _____   BEDTIME: _____   SLEEP (HRS): _____

NOTES FOR THE DAY

_____
_____
_____

IN A STATE OF KETOSIS?

YES   NO   UNSURE

WATER INTAKE TRACKER

FASTING TIMES & DURATION

DAILY ENERGY LEVEL

HIGH	MEDIUM	LOW

1st MEAL

FAT: CARBS: PROTEIN: CALORIES:

EXERCISE / WORKOUT ROUTINE

2nd MEAL

FAT: CARBS: PROTEIN: CALORIES:

Other MEALS & SNACKS

FAT: CARBS: PROTEIN: CALORIES:

TOP 6 PRIORITIES OF THE DAY

END OF THE DAY TOTAL OVERVIEW

FAT	CARBS	PROTEIN	KCAL

MY DAILY PROGRESS **Tracker**

SLEEP TRACKER:

DATE _____

RISE: _____   BEDTIME: _____   SLEEP (HRS): _____

NOTES FOR THE DAY

_____
_____
_____

IN A STATE OF KETOSIS?

YES   NO   UNSURE

WATER INTAKE TRACKER

FASTING TIMES & DURATION

EXERCISE / WORKOUT ROUTINE

	DAILY ENERGY LEVEL	
HIGH	**MEDIUM**	**LOW**

1st MEAL

FAT: CARBS: PROTEIN: CALORIES:

2nd MEAL

FAT: CARBS: PROTEIN: CALORIES:

Other MEALS & SNACKS

FAT: CARBS: PROTEIN: CALORIES:

TOP 6 PRIORITIES OF THE DAY

END OF THE DAY TOTAL OVERVIEW

FAT   CARBS   PROTEIN   KCAL

MY DAILY PROGRESS **Tracker**

SLEEP TRACKER:

DATE _____

RISE: _____

BEDTIME: _____

SLEEP (HRS): _____

NOTES FOR THE DAY

_____

_____

_____

FASTING TIMES & DURATION

EXERCISE / WORKOUT ROUTINE

TOP 6 PRIORITIES OF THE DAY

- ○ _____ ○ _____
- ○ _____ ○ _____
- ○ _____ ○ _____

IN A STATE OF KETOSIS?

YES   NO   UNSURE

WATER INTAKE TRACKER

DAILY ENERGY LEVEL

HIGH	**MEDIUM**	**LOW**

1st MEAL

FAT: CARBS: PROTEIN: CALORIES:

2nd MEAL

FAT: CARBS: PROTEIN: CALORIES:

Other MEALS & SNACKS

FAT: CARBS: PROTEIN: CALORIES:

END OF THE DAY TOTAL OVERVIEW

FAT	CARBS	PROTEIN	KCAL

MEAL Planner

WEEK OF

GROCERY LIST

MON

TUES

WED

THUR

FRI

SAT

SUN

My SHOPPING LIST

FRESH PRODUCE

MEAT AND SEAFOOD

DAIRY PRODUCTS

PANTRY ITEMS

FROZEN / OTHER

MY DAILY PROGRESS **Tracker**

SLEEP TRACKER:

DATE

RISE:

BEDTIME:

SLEEP (HRS):

NOTES FOR THE DAY

IN A STATE OF KETOSIS?

YES   NO   UNSURE

WATER INTAKE TRACKER

FASTING TIMES & DURATION

	DAILY ENERGY LEVEL	
HIGH	**MEDIUM**	**LOW**

1st MEAL

FAT: CARBS: PROTEIN: CALORIES:

EXERCISE / WORKOUT ROUTINE

2nd MEAL

FAT: CARBS: PROTEIN: CALORIES:

Other MEALS & SNACKS

FAT: CARBS: PROTEIN: CALORIES:

TOP 6 PRIORITIES OF THE DAY

END OF THE DAY TOTAL OVERVIEW

FAT   CARBS   PROTEIN   KCAL

MY DAILY PROGRESS **Tracker**

SLEEP TRACKER:

DATE _____

| RISE: | | BEDTIME: | | SLEEP (HRS): |

NOTES FOR THE DAY

_____

_____

_____

FASTING TIMES & DURATION

EXERCISE / WORKOUT ROUTINE

TOP 6 PRIORITIES OF THE DAY

IN A STATE OF KETOSIS?

YES   NO   UNSURE

WATER INTAKE TRACKER

DAILY ENERGY LEVEL		
HIGH	**MEDIUM**	**LOW**

1st MEAL

FAT: CARBS: PROTEIN: CALORIES:

2nd MEAL

FAT: CARBS: PROTEIN: CALORIES:

Other MEALS & SNACKS

FAT: CARBS: PROTEIN: CALORIES:

END OF THE DAY TOTAL OVERVIEW

FAT	CARBS	PROTEIN	KCAL

MY DAILY PROGRESS **Tracker**

SLEEP TRACKER:

DATE

RISE:

BEDTIME:

SLEEP (HRS):

NOTES FOR THE DAY

IN A STATE OF KETOSIS?

YES   NO   UNSURE

WATER INTAKE TRACKER

FASTING TIMES & DURATION

DAILY ENERGY LEVEL		
HIGH	**MEDIUM**	**LOW**

1st MEAL

FAT: CARBS: PROTEIN: CALORIES:

EXERCISE / WORKOUT ROUTINE

2nd MEAL

FAT: CARBS: PROTEIN: CALORIES:

Other MEALS & SNACKS

FAT: CARBS: PROTEIN: CALORIES:

TOP 6 PRIORITIES OF THE DAY

END OF THE DAY TOTAL OVERVIEW

FAT   CARBS   PROTEIN   KCAL

MY DAILY PROGRESS **Tracker**

SLEEP TRACKER:

DATE _____

RISE: _____

BEDTIME: _____

SLEEP (HRS): _____

NOTES FOR THE DAY

_____

_____

_____

FASTING TIMES & DURATION

EXERCISE / WORKOUT ROUTINE

TOP 6 PRIORITIES OF THE DAY

IN A STATE OF KETOSIS?

YES   NO   UNSURE

WATER INTAKE TRACKER

DAILY ENERGY LEVEL

HIGH   **MEDIUM**   **LOW**

1st MEAL

FAT: CARBS: PROTEIN: CALORIES:

2nd MEAL

FAT: CARBS: PROTEIN: CALORIES:

Other MEALS & SNACKS

FAT: CARBS: PROTEIN: CALORIES:

END OF THE DAY TOTAL OVERVIEW

FAT   CARBS   PROTEIN   KCAL

MY DAILY PROGRESS Tracker

SLEEP TRACKER:

DATE _____

RISE: _____   BEDTIME: _____   SLEEP (HRS): _____

NOTES FOR THE DAY

_____

_____

_____

IN A STATE OF KETOSIS?

YES   NO   UNSURE

WATER INTAKE TRACKER

FASTING TIMES & DURATION

EXERCISE / WORKOUT ROUTINE

TOP 6 PRIORITIES OF THE DAY

- _____   - _____
- _____   - _____
- _____   - _____

DAILY ENERGY LEVEL		
HIGH	**MEDIUM**	**LOW**

1st MEAL

FAT: CARBS: PROTEIN: CALORIES:

2nd MEAL

FAT: CARBS: PROTEIN: CALORIES:

Other MEALS & SNACKS

FAT: CARBS: PROTEIN: CALORIES:

END OF THE DAY TOTAL OVERVIEW

FAT   CARBS   PROTEIN   KCAL

MY DAILY PROGRESS **Tracker**

SLEEP TRACKER:

DATE _____

RISE: _____   BEDTIME: _____   SLEEP (HRS): _____

NOTES FOR THE DAY

_____

_____

_____

FASTING TIMES & DURATION

EXERCISE / WORKOUT ROUTINE

TOP 6 PRIORITIES OF THE DAY

IN A STATE OF KETOSIS?

YES   NO   UNSURE

WATER INTAKE TRACKER

DAILY ENERGY LEVEL

HIGH   **MEDIUM**   **LOW**

1st MEAL

FAT: CARBS: PROTEIN: CALORIES:

2nd MEAL

FAT: CARBS: PROTEIN: CALORIES:

Other MEALS & SNACKS

FAT: CARBS: PROTEIN: CALORIES:

END OF THE DAY TOTAL OVERVIEW

FAT   CARBS   PROTEIN   KCAL

MY DAILY PROGRESS **Tracker**

SLEEP TRACKER:

DATE _____

☼ RISE: _____ 🌙 BEDTIME: _____ 💤 SLEEP (HRS): _____

NOTES FOR THE DAY

_____

_____

_____

FASTING TIMES & DURATION

EXERCISE / WORKOUT ROUTINE

TOP 6 PRIORITIES OF THE DAY

⬤ _____   ⬤ _____

⬤ _____   ⬤ _____

⬤ _____   ⬤ _____

IN A STATE OF KETOSIS?

YES   NO   UNSURE

WATER INTAKE TRACKER

DAILY ENERGY LEVEL

HIGH   **MEDIUM**   **LOW**

1st MEAL

FAT: CARBS: PROTEIN: CALORIES:

2nd MEAL

FAT: CARBS: PROTEIN: CALORIES:

Other MEALS & SNACKS

FAT: CARBS: PROTEIN: CALORIES:

END OF THE DAY TOTAL OVERVIEW

FAT   CARBS   PROTEIN   KCAL

MEAL Planner

WEEK OF

GROCERY LIST

MON

TUES

WED

THUR

FRI

SAT

SUN

My SHOPPING LIST

FRESH PRODUCE

MEAT AND SEAFOOD

DAIRY PRODUCTS

PANTRY ITEMS

FROZEN / OTHER

MY DAILY PROGRESS Tracker

SLEEP TRACKER:

DATE _____

RISE: _____ BEDTIME: _____ SLEEP (HRS): _____

NOTES FOR THE DAY

_____
_____
_____

IN A STATE OF KETOSIS?

YES   NO   UNSURE

WATER INTAKE TRACKER

FASTING TIMES & DURATION

DAILY ENERGY LEVEL

HIGH	MEDIUM	LOW

1st MEAL

FAT: CARBS: PROTEIN: CALORIES:

EXERCISE / WORKOUT ROUTINE

2nd MEAL

FAT: CARBS: PROTEIN: CALORIES:

Other MEALS & SNACKS

FAT: CARBS: PROTEIN: CALORIES:

TOP 6 PRIORITIES OF THE DAY

END OF THE DAY TOTAL OVERVIEW

FAT	CARBS	PROTEIN	KCAL

MY DAILY PROGRESS Tracker

SLEEP TRACKER:

DATE _____

RISE: _____

BEDTIME: _____

SLEEP (HRS): _____

NOTES FOR THE DAY

_____

_____

FASTING TIMES & DURATION

EXERCISE / WORKOUT ROUTINE

TOP 6 PRIORITIES OF THE DAY

IN A STATE OF KETOSIS?

YES   NO   UNSURE

WATER INTAKE TRACKER

DAILY ENERGY LEVEL		
HIGH	**MEDIUM**	**LOW**

1st MEAL

FAT: CARBS: PROTEIN: CALORIES:

2nd MEAL

FAT: CARBS: PROTEIN: CALORIES:

Other MEALS & SNACKS

FAT: CARBS: PROTEIN: CALORIES:

END OF THE DAY TOTAL OVERVIEW

FAT   CARBS   PROTEIN   KCAL

MY DAILY PROGRESS **Tracker**

SLEEP TRACKER:

DATE _____

RISE: _____   BEDTIME: _____   SLEEP (HRS): _____

<table>
<tr><td>NOTES FOR THE DAY</td><td>IN A STATE OF KETOSIS?</td></tr>
</table>

NOTES FOR THE DAY

_____

_____

_____

FASTING TIMES & DURATION

EXERCISE / WORKOUT ROUTINE

TOP 6 PRIORITIES OF THE DAY

- ○ _____   ○ _____
- ○ _____   ○ _____
- ○ _____   ○ _____

IN A STATE OF KETOSIS?

YES   NO   UNSURE

WATER INTAKE TRACKER

DAILY ENERGY LEVEL

HIGH   **MEDIUM**   **LOW**

1st MEAL

FAT: CARBS: PROTEIN: CALORIES:

2nd MEAL

FAT: CARBS: PROTEIN: CALORIES:

Other MEALS & SNACKS

FAT: CARBS: PROTEIN: CALORIES:

END OF THE DAY TOTAL OVERVIEW

FAT   CARBS   PROTEIN   KCAL

MY DAILY PROGRESS **Tracker**

SLEEP TRACKER:

DATE _____

| RISE: | BEDTIME: | SLEEP (HRS): |

NOTES FOR THE DAY

IN A STATE OF KETOSIS?

YES   NO   UNSURE

WATER INTAKE TRACKER

FASTING TIMES & DURATION

| DAILY ENERGY LEVEL |
| **HIGH**   **MEDIUM**   **LOW** |

1st MEAL

FAT: CARBS: PROTEIN: CALORIES:

EXERCISE / WORKOUT ROUTINE

2nd MEAL

FAT: CARBS: PROTEIN: CALORIES:

Other MEALS & SNACKS

FAT: CARBS: PROTEIN: CALORIES:

TOP 6 PRIORITIES OF THE DAY

END OF THE DAY TOTAL OVERVIEW

FAT   CARBS   PROTEIN   KCAL

MY DAILY PROGRESS **Tracker**

SLEEP TRACKER:

DATE _____

RISE: _____

BEDTIME: _____

SLEEP (HRS): _____

NOTES FOR THE DAY

_____
_____
_____

FASTING TIMES & DURATION

EXERCISE / WORKOUT ROUTINE

TOP 6 PRIORITIES OF THE DAY

IN A STATE OF KETOSIS?

YES   NO   UNSURE

WATER INTAKE TRACKER

DAILY ENERGY LEVEL

HIGH   **MEDIUM**   **LOW**

1st MEAL

FAT: CARBS: PROTEIN: CALORIES:

2nd MEAL

FAT: CARBS: PROTEIN: CALORIES:

Other MEALS & SNACKS

FAT: CARBS: PROTEIN: CALORIES:

END OF THE DAY TOTAL OVERVIEW

FAT   CARBS   PROTEIN   KCAL

MY DAILY PROGRESS **Tracker**

SLEEP TRACKER:

DATE _____

RISE: _____

BEDTIME: _____

SLEEP (HRS): _____

NOTES FOR THE DAY

_____
_____
_____

IN A STATE OF KETOSIS?

YES   NO   UNSURE

WATER INTAKE TRACKER

FASTING TIMES & DURATION

DAILY ENERGY LEVEL

HIGH   **MEDIUM**   **LOW**

1st **MEAL**

FAT: CARBS: PROTEIN: CALORIES:

EXERCISE / WORKOUT ROUTINE

2nd **MEAL**

FAT: CARBS: PROTEIN: CALORIES:

Other **MEALS** & **SNACKS**

FAT: CARBS: PROTEIN: CALORIES:

TOP 6 PRIORITIES OF THE DAY

END OF THE DAY TOTAL OVERVIEW

FAT   CARBS   PROTEIN   KCAL

MY DAILY PROGRESS **Tracker**

SLEEP TRACKER:

DATE _____

RISE: _____   BEDTIME: _____   SLEEP (HRS): _____

NOTES FOR THE DAY

_____

_____

_____

IN A STATE OF KETOSIS?

YES   NO   UNSURE

WATER INTAKE TRACKER

FASTING TIMES & DURATION

DAILY ENERGY LEVEL

HIGH   **MEDIUM**   **LOW**

1st MEAL

FAT: CARBS: PROTEIN: CALORIES:

2nd MEAL

FAT: CARBS: PROTEIN: CALORIES:

EXERCISE / WORKOUT ROUTINE

Other MEALS & SNACKS

FAT: CARBS: PROTEIN: CALORIES:

TOP 6 PRIORITIES OF THE DAY

END OF THE DAY TOTAL OVERVIEW

FAT   CARBS   PROTEIN   KCAL

MEAL **Planner**

WEEK OF

GROCERY LIST

- [ ]
- [ ]
- [ ]
- [ ]
- [ ]
- [ ]
- [ ]
- [ ]
- [ ]
- [ ]
- [ ]
- [ ]
- [ ]
- [ ]
- [ ]
- [ ]
- [ ]

MON

TUES

WED

THUR

FRI

SAT

SUN

My SHOPPING LIST

FRESH PRODUCE

MEAT AND SEAFOOD

DAIRY PRODUCTS

PANTRY ITEMS

FROZEN / OTHER

MY DAILY PROGRESS **Tracker**

SLEEP TRACKER:

DATE

RISE:

BEDTIME:

SLEEP (HRS):

NOTES FOR THE DAY

IN A STATE OF KETOSIS?

YES   NO   UNSURE

WATER INTAKE TRACKER

FASTING TIMES & DURATION

DAILY ENERGY LEVEL		
HIGH	**MEDIUM**	**LOW**

1st MEAL

FAT: CARBS: PROTEIN: CALORIES:

EXERCISE / WORKOUT ROUTINE

2nd MEAL

FAT: CARBS: PROTEIN: CALORIES:

Other MEALS & SNACKS

FAT: CARBS: PROTEIN: CALORIES:

TOP 6 PRIORITIES OF THE DAY

END OF THE DAY TOTAL OVERVIEW

FAT   CARBS   PROTEIN   KCAL

MY DAILY PROGRESS **Tracker**

SLEEP TRACKER:

DATE _____

RISE: _____   BEDTIME: _____   SLEEP (HRS): _____

NOTES FOR THE DAY

_____

_____

_____

IN A STATE OF KETOSIS?

YES   NO   UNSURE

WATER INTAKE TRACKER

FASTING TIMES & DURATION

DAILY ENERGY LEVEL ·

HIGH	MEDIUM	LOW

1st MEAL

FAT: CARBS: PROTEIN: CALORIES:

EXERCISE / WORKOUT ROUTINE

2nd MEAL

FAT: CARBS: PROTEIN: CALORIES:

Other MEALS & SNACKS

FAT: CARBS: PROTEIN: CALORIES:

TOP 6 PRIORITIES OF THE DAY

- ⊙ _____   ⊙ _____
- ⊙ _____   ⊙ _____
- ⊙ _____   ⊙ _____

END OF THE DAY TOTAL OVERVIEW

FAT   CARBS   PROTEIN   KCAL

MY DAILY PROGRESS **Tracker**

SLEEP TRACKER:

DATE _____

RISE: _____   BEDTIME: _____   SLEEP (HRS): _____

NOTES FOR THE DAY
_____
_____
_____

FASTING TIMES & DURATION

EXERCISE / WORKOUT ROUTINE

TOP 6 PRIORITIES OF THE DAY
○ _____   ○ _____
○ _____   ○ _____
○ _____   ○ _____

IN A STATE OF KETOSIS?

YES   NO   UNSURE

WATER INTAKE TRACKER

DAILY ENERGY LEVEL

HIGH   **MEDIUM**   **LOW**

1st MEAL

FAT: CARBS: PROTEIN: CALORIES:

2nd MEAL

FAT: CARBS: PROTEIN: CALORIES:

Other MEALS & SNACKS

FAT: CARBS: PROTEIN: CALORIES:

END OF THE DAY TOTAL OVERVIEW

FAT   CARBS   PROTEIN   KCAL

MY DAILY PROGRESS **Tracker**

SLEEP TRACKER:

DATE _____

RISE: _____

BEDTIME: _____

SLEEP (HRS): _____

NOTES FOR THE DAY

_____
_____
_____

IN A STATE OF KETOSIS?

YES   NO   UNSURE

WATER INTAKE TRACKER

FASTING TIMES & DURATION

DAILY ENERGY LEVEL		
HIGH	**MEDIUM**	**LOW**

1st MEAL

FAT: CARBS: PROTEIN: CALORIES:

EXERCISE / WORKOUT ROUTINE

2nd MEAL

FAT: CARBS: PROTEIN: CALORIES:

Other MEALS & SNACKS

FAT: CARBS: PROTEIN: CALORIES:

TOP 6 PRIORITIES OF THE DAY

END OF THE DAY TOTAL OVERVIEW

FAT	CARBS	PROTEIN	KCAL

MY DAILY PROGRESS **Tracker**

SLEEP TRACKER:

DATE _____

RISE: _____ BEDTIME: _____ SLEEP (HRS): _____

NOTES FOR THE DAY

_____

_____

_____

IN A STATE OF KETOSIS?

YES   NO   UNSURE

WATER INTAKE TRACKER

FASTING TIMES & DURATION

DAILY ENERGY LEVEL

HIGH	MEDIUM	LOW

1st MEAL

FAT: CARBS: PROTEIN: CALORIES:

2nd MEAL

FAT: CARBS: PROTEIN: CALORIES:

EXERCISE / WORKOUT ROUTINE

Other MEALS & SNACKS

FAT: CARBS: PROTEIN: CALORIES:

TOP 6 PRIORITIES OF THE DAY

- _____ _____
- _____ _____
- _____ _____

END OF THE DAY TOTAL OVERVIEW

FAT   CARBS   PROTEIN   KCAL

MY DAILY PROGRESS **Tracker**

SLEEP TRACKER:

DATE _____

RISE: _____   BEDTIME: _____   SLEEP (HRS): _____

NOTES FOR THE DAY

_____
_____
_____

FASTING TIMES & DURATION

EXERCISE / WORKOUT ROUTINE

TOP 6 PRIORITIES OF THE DAY

IN A STATE OF KETOSIS?

YES   NO   UNSURE

WATER INTAKE TRACKER

DAILY ENERGY LEVEL

HIGH   **MEDIUM**   **LOW**

1st MEAL

FAT: CARBS: PROTEIN: CALORIES:

2nd MEAL

FAT: CARBS: PROTEIN: CALORIES:

Other MEALS & SNACKS

FAT: CARBS: PROTEIN: CALORIES:

END OF THE DAY TOTAL OVERVIEW

FAT   CARBS   PROTEIN   KCAL

MY DAILY PROGRESS **Tracker**

SLEEP TRACKER:

DATE _____

RISE: _____   BEDTIME: _____   SLEEP (HRS): _____

NOTES FOR THE DAY

_____

_____

_____

IN A STATE OF KETOSIS?

YES   NO   UNSURE

WATER INTAKE TRACKER

FASTING TIMES & DURATION

DAILY ENERGY LEVEL

HIGH   **MEDIUM**   **LOW**

1st MEAL

FAT: CARBS: PROTEIN: CALORIES:

EXERCISE / WORKOUT ROUTINE

2nd MEAL

FAT: CARBS: PROTEIN: CALORIES:

Other MEALS & SNACKS

FAT: CARBS: PROTEIN: CALORIES:

TOP 6 PRIORITIES OF THE DAY

END OF THE DAY TOTAL OVERVIEW

FAT   CARBS   PROTEIN   KCAL

WEIGHT LOSS End Date

What are some of your thoughts about your 90-Day Keto Journey?

Do you plan to continue doing Keto? What will you do differently? What will you do more of?

PERSONAL MILESTONES

WEIGHT LOSS **Results**

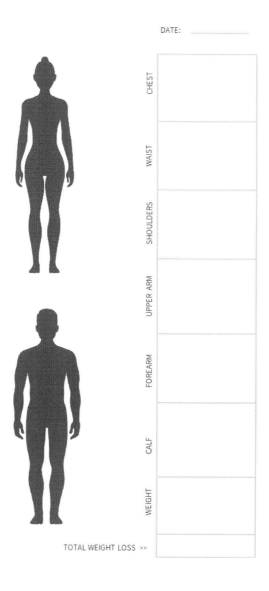

DATE:

	CHEST	
	WAIST	
	SHOULDERS	
	UPPER ARM	
	FOREARM	
	CALF	
	WEIGHT	
TOTAL WEIGHT LOSS >>		

My **Recipes**

RECIPE NAME:

	Keto	Low Carb	Paleo	Vegetarian	Vegan	Dairy Free	Gluten Free
	☐	☐	☐	☐	☐	☐	☐

QTY	INGREDIENTS	RECIPE INSTRUCTIONS

NOTES & RECIPE REVIEW

Serves	
Prep Time	
Cook Time	
Tools	
Temp	

Total	Carbs	Fat	Protein	Cals

My **Recipes**

RECIPE NAME:

Keto	Low Carb	Paleo	Vegetarian	Vegan	Dairy Free	Gluten Free
☐	☐	☐	☐	☐	☐	☐

QTY	INGREDIENTS	RECIPE INSTRUCTIONS

NOTES & RECIPE REVIEW

Serves	
Prep Time	
Cook Time	
Tools	
Temp	

Total	Carbs	Fat	Protein	Cals

My **Recipes**

RECIPE NAME:

	Keto	Low Carb	Paleo	Vegetarian	Vegan	Dairy Free	Gluten Free
	☐	☐	☐	☐	☐	☐	☐

QTY	INGREDIENTS	RECIPE INSTRUCTIONS

NOTES & RECIPE REVIEW		

Serves	
Prep Time	
Cook Time	
Tools	
Temp	

Total	Carbs	Fat	Protein	Cals

My **Recipes**

RECIPE NAME:

	Keto	Low Carb	Paleo	Vegetarian	Vegan	Dairy Free	Gluten Free
	☐	☐	☐	☐	☐	☐	☐

QTY	INGREDIENTS	RECIPE INSTRUCTIONS

NOTES & RECIPE REVIEW		Serves	
		Prep Time	
		Cook Time	
		Tools	
		Temp	

Total	Carbs	Fat	Protein	Cals

My **Recipes**

RECIPE NAME:

	Keto	Low Carb	Paleo	Vegetarian	Vegan	Dairy Free	Gluten Free
	☐	☐	☐	☐	☐	☐	☐

QTY	INGREDIENTS	RECIPE INSTRUCTIONS

NOTES & RECIPE REVIEW	

Serves	
Prep Time	
Cook Time	
Tools	
Temp	

Total	Carbs	Fat	Protein	Cals

My **Recipes**

RECIPE NAME:

	Keto	Low Carb	Paleo	Vegetarian	Vegan	Dairy Free	Gluten Free
	☐	☐	☐	☐	☐	☐	☐

QTY	INGREDIENTS	RECIPE INSTRUCTIONS

NOTES & RECIPE REVIEW		

Serves	
Prep Time	
Cook Time	
Tools	
Temp	

Total	Carbs	Fat	Protein	Cals

My **Recipes**

RECIPE NAME:

Keto	Low Carb	Paleo	Vegetarian	Vegan	Dairy Free	Gluten Free
☐	☐	☐	☐	☐	☐	☐

QTY	INGREDIENTS	RECIPE INSTRUCTIONS

NOTES & RECIPE REVIEW

Serves	
Prep Time	
Cook Time	
Tools	
Temp	

Total	Carbs	Fat	Protein	Cals

My **Recipes**

RECIPE NAME:

	Keto	Low Carb	Paleo	Vegetarian	Vegan	Dairy Free	Gluten Free
	☐	☐	☐	☐	☐	☐	☐

QTY	INGREDIENTS	RECIPE INSTRUCTIONS

NOTES & RECIPE REVIEW

Serves	
Prep Time	
Cook Time	
Tools	
Temp	

Total	Carbs	Fat	Protein	Cals

My **Recipes**

RECIPE NAME:

	Keto	Low Carb	Paleo	Vegetarian	Vegan	Dairy Free	Gluten Free
	☐	☐	☐	☐	☐	☐	☐

QTY	INGREDIENTS	RECIPE INSTRUCTIONS

NOTES & RECIPE REVIEW

Serves	
Prep Time	
Cook Time	
Tools	
Temp	

Total	Carbs	Fat	Protein	Cals

My **Recipes**

RECIPE NAME:

Keto	Low Carb	Paleo	Vegetarian	Vegan	Dairy Free	Gluten Free
☐	☐	☐	☐	☐	☐	☐

QTY	INGREDIENTS

RECIPE INSTRUCTIONS

NOTES & RECIPE REVIEW

Serves	
Prep Time	
Cook Time	
Tools	
Temp	

Total	Carbs	Fat	Protein	Cals

Made in the USA
Las Vegas, NV
17 February 2023

67676494R00085